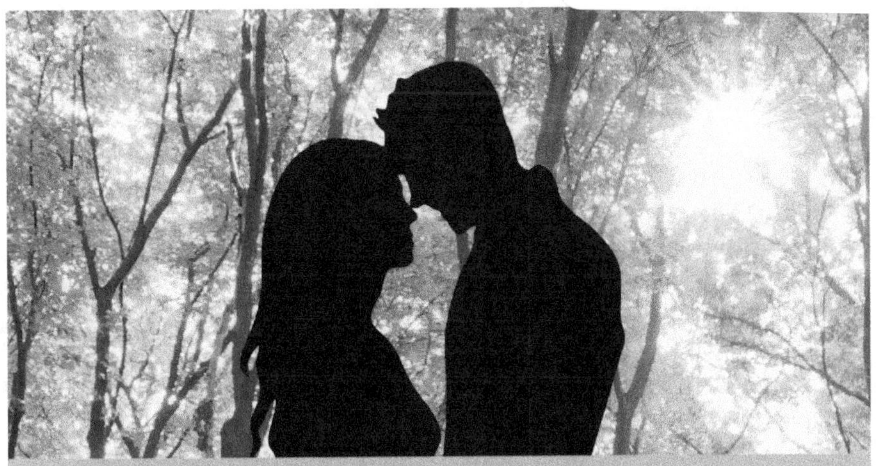

SEXUAL WELLNESS

Optimize Your Relationship, Pleasure, and Sexual Health

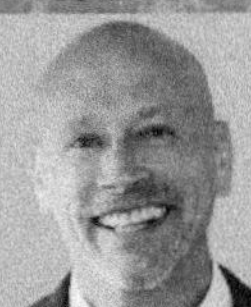

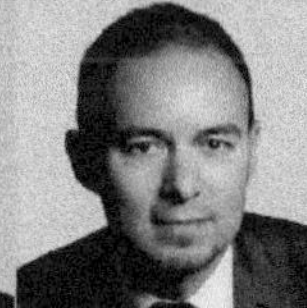

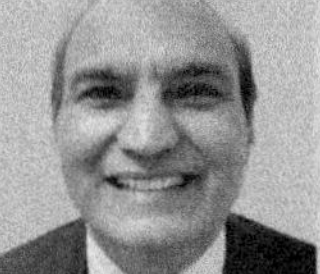

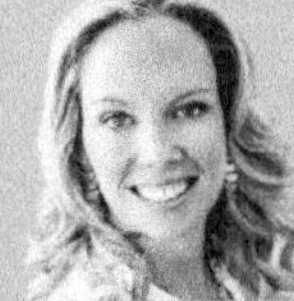

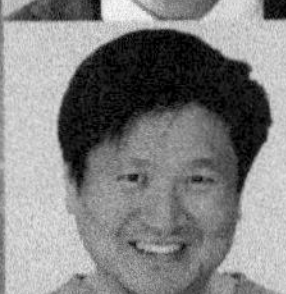
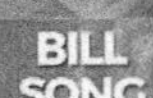

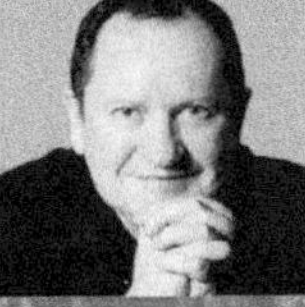

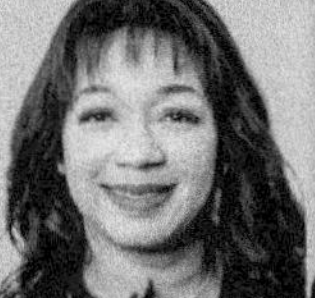

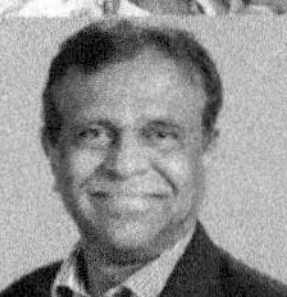

Sexual Wellness: Optimize Your Relationship, Pleasure & Sexual Health

Leave a review on Amazon: SexualWellnessBook.com/amazon
Free gift from Dr. Charles Runels: SexualWellnessBook.com/gift

**Chapter 7:
Recover Your Sex Life
After Prostate Cancer
with Dr. Ramesh Kumar**

Introduction:
What This Book Can Do for You

I assembled the authors of this book to share their ideas and advice and knowledge with a single objective in mind: to help you enjoy more sexual pleasure and deeper, stronger love relations through better sexual health and wellness.

This is no idle goal. Anyone at any age can enjoy better sex. Moreover, you owe it to yourself, and to your family to learn and to practice ways to better sex.

When I use the word "sex," I draw a large circle and mean all of the following: touch, erotic words, and (of course) genitals touching genitals and engorged with the touching; but, also, I mean a body filled with desire and pleasure and sensation and inspiration; I mean the building, the plateau, and the orgasm (all of it, and no part of it better than another); I mean hair and breasts and skin, mouths, genitals, hands; I mean every part of the body awake and alive and more alive because of the sexual urge, and because of the mechanical, emotional and physiological release of that urge; moreover, and (just as importantly) I mean the transmutation of that urge into creativity and energy and productivity and personality and caring and courage and love and prayer.

Sex is much more than genitals touching genitals.

And, sex, thought of in this way, is very important—even if you live alone.

The sexual urge gives sparkle to personality, fervor to prayer, and determination to commerce. **Napoleon Hill** said, in *Think & Grow Rich*, that the transmutation of sexual energy into creative, productive, and profitable work is the primary force behind most great fortunes.

Reiner Maria Rilke said, in Letters to a Young Poet, that creativity is directly related to the sexual urge.

The transmutation of sexual energy into prayer that connects with a higher power should be the idea behind the celibacy, when chosen, of the priests of any true scripture.

Sex is much more than genitals touching genitals. Sex deserves your attention and in this book, the authors give you specific ideas to make both your sex and your life better.

Susan, a seventy-two year-old woman, had just put her wife in the nursing home when she came as a patient to see me. One day, in my office, she said, "I live alone, but I make love to myself! Why should men have all the fun? Because of the treatment you gave me, my orgasms are stronger. I sleep better after masturbation. And, I sell more at work when I enjoy a strong sex drive."

Susan's story is very common with mature women. On the other hand, when sex is not functioning, I've observed by speaking with thousands of people in my office, sexual brokenness can strain marriages beyond repair— leading to divorce and to parents living separated from each other *and from their children. In this way, good sexual function with your partner indirectly supports the nurturing of your children.*

Sex and orgasm facilitate a spiritual and emotional bond between two people that comes with much more difficulty without sex.

Emerson called *"beauty"* the "scaffolding of love." He could have more specifically said that *"sex* is the scaffolding of love."

Of course, deep love relations can happen without the bodily functions that most consider to be sex. But, just as it is much more difficult to build a house without scaffolding, it is also difficult to build a romantic love relationship without sex.

The purpose of this book is to help you too expand your view of what sex is and to help you on the path to better sexual wellness and to deeper relations.

After over twenty-five years of caring for men and women as their physician, I have seen first hand the anhedonic, flat facial expressions of those who mechanically live their life without the pleasure and the creativity of good sex.

Brenda sat in my office and told me that she wanted to lose forty pounds. She also suffered with mild depression and anxiety, fatigue, and complained of "foggy" thinking.

When I asked her about her sexual wellness, she said, "I am divorced and am perfectly happy with not having to bother with a sex drive. I just want to lose weight and have more energy."

I said to her, "I would never say that your low sex drive is a problem if you prefer to live without sex.

Still, I should warn you that if I do what I know to do to help you lose weight, increase your energy, and clear the fog in your brain—as a side effect, you will want to have sex."

Seven weeks later, when Brenda came back to see me after treatment, I could see when she walked into the room that things were much different with her. She smiled more than when we first met, her clothes were new and smaller, and her speech was quicker and warmer.

She started talking excitedly before she sat down, "I'm dating an amazing man. He's kind to me and to my children, but mostly I'm just having more fun. I didn't miss sex before your treatment, but now with this new sex drive, I'm just enjoying life more at work and at home— even when not having sex!"

"Is that strange?" she asked.

It's not strange at all. ***Sex is about much more that what happens in the bedroom.***

Brenda's story brings up an important fact about women's sex: to be diagnosed as having sexual dysfunction, a woman must be psychologically distressed about her sex life. In contrast, for example, if a man cannot achieve a firm erection— whether or not he is psychologically bothered— he has a sexual disorder, erectile dysfunction.

But, if a woman cannot achieve orgasm or suffers with painful sex, or has no libido, and if that woman is not psychologically distressed by the situation, she does NOT have sexual dysfunction. *This difference in definitions between men and women could explain why sexual dysfunction is more common in older men and in YOUNGER women!* Older women are less likely than younger women to be emotionally distressed by dyspareunia, and decreased orgasm, or decreased libido; so, the older women are not counted.

Again, the older women are simply not counted because they sometimes quit complaining.

Still, even with this strict definition of sexual dysfunction, around forty percent of women suffer with sexual problems and about the same number of men (more in men older than fifty years old).

In summary, around forty percent of women (even more in younger women) and a similar number of men (even more in older men) suffers distress about their sex life. That means that close to one half of all adults suffer not only the problems of broken sex but also the associated problems of strained or broken relationships, decreased creativity, sleep disturbance, decreased energy, foggy thinking, decreased job performance, depression, and just plain loss of fun even when doing what should be fun.

So, thinking and talking and reading about sex is very important and should be done much more than it is.

Congratulations for having the courage to make things better by improving your sexual wellness. Just as you can improve health and vitality even when you are not sick, you can improve sexual health and vitality at any age— even if sex is already very good.

Why Another Book About Sex?

With thousands of popular books, and science and medical textbooks about sex, why write another one?

First, we produced this book because the science changes so fast that an updated book with contributions by practicing physicians who also understand the most up-to-date science was needed. The second reason (covered in the Prologue) is that an emphasis on a "Systems Approach" is needed.

The Seven Authors of This Book

Here, in this book you'll find the collective advice of seven separate physicians who understand the most up-to-date science but also bring to that science more than 100 years of collective experience in taking care of people seeking to make sex better. Each of the seven contributors have cared for thousands of people both well and not well to help them find better sex.

In Chapter 1, **Dr. Jean Luc Le Provost** describes powerful but simple daily routines that can be used to improve overall health in such a way to specifically improve sexual wellness.

In Chapter 2, **Dr. Prabhat Soni,** uses his vast experience as a pulmonologist and sleep specialist to show you ways to optimize sleep and why poor sleep can kill your sex life. You need a functioning brain to have sex. But, just as importantly, the pituitary gland is literally attached to that brain, controls all the other glands, and is profoundly affected by sleep.

Dr. Cristyn Watkins, in Chapter 3, discusses her personal battles and how out of those battles she became an expert in cellular therapies that improve sexual wellness from the level of tissue and histology. Healthy tissue makes for healthy, fully functioning genitalia.

In Chapter 4, ***Dr. Bill Song*** discusses a number of options to help increase the size of the penis— for improved confidence in men and enhanced pleasure for their lovers. Multiple modalities can be used. He helps you sort the options.

In Chapter 5, ***Dr. Dan Botha*** discusses extremely helpful new technology that helps with a more exact treatment of erectile dysfunction and of Peyronie's disease. No more guessing where the problem is or if and how things might be improving after treatment.

In Chapter 6, ***Dr. Kimberly Evans*** describes how in her practice of gynecology she improves sexual wellness and pleasure by expertly micromanaging the hormones of women and their partners. Hormones affect the growth and function of every body tissue; so there's no finding your best sexual wellness without this step.

And finally, in Chapter 7, **Dr. Ramesh Kumar** draws from his decades of experience as a radiation oncologist to describe ways to recover sexual desire, health, and pleasure after cancer— especially prostate cancer.

Final Words

Good sexual health, like good health in general is not an event where you do one or two things occasionally and all is good for the rest of your life. Wellness, sexual or otherwise, arises with the ***daily practice*** of certain behaviors combined with specific modern therapies when things are broken.

Please consider this book a guide to your better sexual wellness but also recognize that as your body changes and as science advances, your practices should also change. So, I invite you to stay in touch with me and with the authors of this book. Subscribe to our emails at <u>SexualWellnessBook.com</u> to stay informed of the latest and best treatments and practices (and for free offers available only to the buyers of this book).

If you'd like more assistance, contact any of the authors of this book and ask your own physician about the topics covered.

After you've had a chance to read this volume and to begin implementing what you've learned (always with the guidance of your personal physician), I hope you'll contact me to let me know how you're doing.

Not only will you benefit greatly from the information in this book; but, by your renewed vitality, so will your family, your friends, your business, and possibly your soul satisfaction.

Write to me soon! I love to hear good news— especially when I may have contributed in a small way.

Your fellow sojourner,

Charles

Charles Runels MD

Charles Runels, MD

Fairhope, AL
November 2020

Leave a review of this book on Amazon:
SexualWellnessBook.com/amazon

*P.S. To understand the framework **needed to intelligently plan your own personal, tailor-made steps to better sex,** please be sure to turn the page and read the* **"Prologue: The Orgasm System."**

Prologue:
The Orgasm System
by Dr. Charles Runels

As a child, probably in about sixth grade, your teacher taught you to draw the respiratory system, the gastrointestinal system, and the reproductive system. Why were you taught to draw on the same piece of paper the ovaries, the cervix, and fallopian tubes (and call it the "reproductive system")? And then, on another piece of paper, why did you draw the stomach, the esophagus, and the small intestines (and call it the "gastrointestinal system")?

You were taught to think in terms of "systems" because looking only at individual parts— in isolation— will not give an understanding of how the parts work together to accomplish a purpose. Multiple parts working together to accomplish one purpose makes a "system."

For an example of the importance of systems analysis, consider what happens if you take your car to a mechanic because the engine sputters. The mechanic would use systems analysis to fix your car. Thinking about each part of the system, could the gasoline line be clogged? It could be a spark plug isn't firing. The electronic fuel injector may not be firing. The car may just be out of gas. Without knowing about all of those parts of the fuel system and how the parts work together, a mechanic could neither repair a broken fuel system nor optimize a working system.

A mechanic who boasted of being an expert at fuel lines but possessed no understanding or consideration of the whole system would not be capable of optimizing or repairing the fuel system except when lucky enough to be repairing someone's car that happens to have a clogged fuel line.

The classic metaphor is that if you have a hammer then everything looks like a nail. Be careful when healthcare providers or sex therapists think in terms of everything being the nail that matches their hammer.

To apply that same idea to the body (so that we can understand orgasm), first, consider the respiratory system. The parts of the respiratory system, working together, supply oxygen to the cells of the body and remove carbon dioxide. If the system malfunctions, the person feels short of breath. If the system fails, then the person dies from asphyxiation/suffocation. Parts of the system include the trachea, bronchial tubes, the alveoli, and the red blood cells (in the circulatory system) which carry the oxygen, and the diaphragm that expands the lungs and moves air in and out. You probably remember drawing the system as a child.

Knowing or thinking about only one part of that system would not allow the most effective cure. Just as importantly, if you could breathe normally, but you want your breathing to function in a superior way (as an Olympic athlete), then you could use your knowledge of the same systems analysis to turn up the average system to create a superior respiratory system.

For example, as an endurance athlete wanting to not feel short of breath, even when running fast in a long distance, you could train in Denver, Colorado, where your adaptation to the altitude would increase the number of red blood cells to give you extra oxygen-carrying ability. Then when you compete at sea level you will be able to run faster and farther without crossing your anaerobic threshold and suffering lactic acid build up and fatigue.

So, to either repair a broken system or to improve the functioning system, a pulmonologist needs to know not just about each individual part, but also how the parts work together. This consideration of how all the parts work together, Systems Analysis, is by far the best way to find a path to healing and to help find your best functioning— far above just being well.

We have a need for systems analysis for anything from a car to breathing, to digesting our food, to reproduction, to orgasm.

The Reproductive System is Not the Orgasm System

The reproductive system is not the same as the orgasm system. You can reproduce without an orgasm. Ten percent of women never experience an orgasm, but many of them still deliver children. You can also have an orgasm without becoming pregnant.

So reproduction and sexual pleasure/orgasm are not the same. The organs involved in the two processes differ. Even when the anatomical organs involved in those two processes overlap, the individual organs can function differently when the goal is orgasm and pleasure compared to when the goal is reproduction.

Also, the way components of the two systems work together differs between reproduction and orgasm (sexual pleasure).

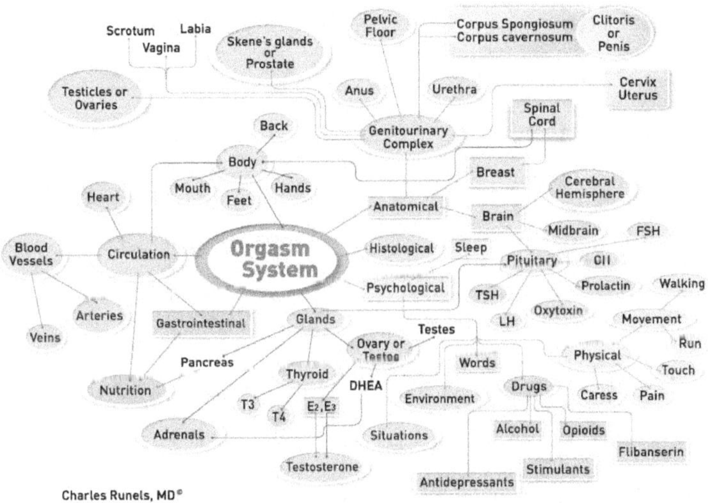

I've seen posters and read books that explain the nervous system and the respiratory system and the cardiovascular system and the gastrointestinal system and the reproductive system. But, I've never seen anyone explain to my satisfaction the Orgasm System or draw a diagram that could be put on a poster to explain the system. Because the system of orgasm is neither as widely taught nor understood as the other body systems, when men and women struggle with sex, they often receive the "hammer" that her consultant wields (thinking the problem must be the *matching-nail-latest-drug-or-device*) without a strategic consideration of the entire system.

For example, if a woman goes to the cashier at the sex toy store, then the cashier sells the woman a vibrator and so improves the sensation of the stimulation of the genital-urinary system; but, maybe that's not the problem. Maybe the woman enjoys a very sensitive clitoral complex but suffers with a hormonal problem— for example, a very low testosterone level.

On the other hand, if the woman goes to the psychotherapist or a family counselor who's trying to help her achieve orgasm, the therapist may recommend sensate focus or perhaps counseling about what happened with the woman as a child. But, maybe the woman suffers with a clitoral hood that's phimosed by lichen sclerosus so that it can't be retracted— the clitoris cannot be seen nor stimulated because of scarring. So, the psychotherapy may help her live more happily with the problem; but, if the woman wants the problem to go away, then she needs a surgical intervention with re-exposure of the clitoris and then treatment of her lichen sclerosus with topical steroids or with the O-Shot® procedure.

As a more familiar example, back to the respiratory system, if you give someone bronchial dilators to help with shortness of breath, but the real problem is not bronchospasm but an extreme paucity of red blood cells (T9 carry the oxygen) from B12 deficiency, then you turn shortness-of-breath-from-bronchospasm into your nail because you have a "bronchodilators hammer." Pulmonologists do not make that mistake in the respiratory world because they are taught to meticulously think in terms of systems analysis. But the healer with a hammer turning most every patient's sexual dysfunction into a nail can be spotted much too often in the world of sexual dysfunction.

For example, much too often, I've seen women who were treated for decreased sex drive with vibrators and KY Jelly when the woman suffered from a treatable specific etiology that broke the orgasm system like testosterone deficiency, or elevated prolactin from a pituitary adenoma, or from decreased sensation from nerve damage from riding a bicycle or from diabetes.

There Are No Magic Bullets

So, as you read through this book, and then consider what you read with your physician and health care team, remember to consider the whole system. There may only be one component that needs attention, but more likely you'll find your best sexual pleasure and best relationships if you consider the whole system and embark on a life-long journey to continually find the best health for all components of the system.

Being well, being sexually well, is a life-long, artful, strategic, spiritual, healthful, courageous pursuit—not a one time event.

The Orgasm System Works Even Without Orgasm

Even without orgasm, the pursuit of pleasure and reaching the edge of orgasm, brings much energy. In fact, many have argued that getting near orgasm without spilling over into orgasm can bring the most benefits.

The energy, the desire, the clarity, the courage that comes with desire can sometimes be dissipated, especially in men, by the orgasm itself. But, the desire that leads to orgasm can be ridden, surfed like a wave, to bring courage, genius, romance, and creativity. The Sutras, the Dao, Thoreau, Freud, Franklin are just a few of the places where you'll find this surfing discussed (using different words but all discussing the same phenomenon).

So, it's important to consider that the Orgasm System brings great benefit without orgasm. For further discussion of this idea, please see my book, Anytime…for as Long as You Want: Strength, Genius, Libido, & Erection by Integrative Sex Transmutation by going to SexualWellnessBook.com/anytime.

The Orgasm Also Works Well When You Experience Orgasm

An orgasm resets your brain like pushing the "reboot" button resets your computer. Scientists don't fully understand the changes that occur (with your brain rebooted by orgasm); but, we know the explosion of biochemical and physiological changes that occur with orgasm dramatically alters brain function. With orgasm you can improve your sense of well-being, your creativity, sleep, energy, peace of mind, your feelings about the situation, and the person surrounding your orgasm.

As an example of the profound effects of orgasm, consider that research shows that when heterosexual men (with no previous experience of homosexuality), become trapped on a Navy ship with other men for an extended time, they sometimes turn to other men for sexual release. Then when these previously heterosexual men leave the ship, because they experienced orgasm with other men, they become psychologically bonded to the idea of men as an erotic foundation and can remain homosexually inclined for the remainder of their life after leaving the ship. Orgasm causes the man to become attached to the partner in orgasm.

If you apply that same idea to the marriage bed, the implications become profound. Orgasm serves not only to bring you pleasure and perhaps to facilitate procreation (by helping encourage repeated copulation/insemination and to propel sperm to the egg with muscular contractions)— orgasm also serves to develop and to sustain deep relationships by connecting you emotionally to your lover.

The cascade effect of orgasm followed by connection then fuels your happiness machine— family and love relations. Good orgasms can help keep mother and father living happily together under the same roof with the children. Good orgasm can help you reveal your secret self to your partner's view so that you feel loved instead of feeling your lover only views and loves your mask.

The feeling of not being seen and known leads to loneliness—even when naked in bed, even after bearing children. Orgasm helps you remove the mask to be loved for what's beneath. Your lover's participation in your orgasm becomes the magic spectacles that help you find love by seeing each other.

The deepening relationship that happens with orgasm occurs not only with your lover but also with yourself. Many women who choose to live alone have told me that they make love to themselves.

Orgasm brings much more than erotic pleasure. Ironically, even though orgasm does bring pleasure, if the purpose of orgasm becomes only about pleasure, then orgasm becomes more difficult and frustrating to find. The most amazing orgasms, with all of the splendid secondary effects, usually come when orgasm ceases to be your goal.

That idea— finding something by ceasing to strive for it— could confuse or frustrate you. But relax, because when you understand the orgasm system by study and by applying what you learn here, then you can enjoy the process of optimizing each part of the system. Then, you will not only enjoy more intense sexual pleasure, but also will find better health and an expansion of your life. Congratulations for having the courage to make the journey.

For the past 30 years, as a physician, I personally conducted detailed interviews and blood analysis and careful treatment of over 5,000 men and women for their sexual and overall health— thinking deeply about both their sexuality, their hormones, and their overall health. I've published research and books on the orgasmic response, and invented procedures (the O-Shot® and the P-Shot®) to help women and men heal the genital tissue. I trained hundreds of physicians in over 50 countries to better help women with the sexual response. I've lectured to physicians in Greece, Spain, Serbia, India, New Zealand, Canada, the United Kingdom, Australia, Italy, and throughout the US and other countries.

I've interviewed and cared for men and women who are attorneys, porn stars, Playboy Bunnies, nuns, preachers, mothers, grandmothers, teachers, sex educators, gynecologists, urologists, Baptists, Hindu, Muslim, Jewish, professors, students, prostitutes, the anorgasmic and the hypersexual, the monogamous and the polyamorous.

If I haven't learned a few things from that many people, I'd need to be very distracted. So, I hope you'll trust me enough to at least report to you for your consideration a few of my observations and suggestions.

I'm only telling you my personal opinions and observations and the relevant research. For your personal situation, nothing substitutes for a private consultation with your own physician. Still, I hope that what you find in this book will help you and your physician move more expertly, quickly, and thoughtfully into the journey to your best sexual health.

Unfortunately, research shows that most women (86%) never converse with their physician about sex even though around 40% of women experience emotional distress about their sexual function and even though almost all women desire to improve their sex. Research also shows that when women bring up the subject of sex, most physicians change the subject after the first questions— with no significant conversation or resolution. Hopefully, with your new knowledge of the intricacies of the orgasm system, you can help facilitate the conversation and the journey to your best sex.

Should your physician seem reluctant to help you, then try one time to use your knowledge and understanding of the orgasm system that you learn here to force the conversation. If you still feel as if your physician will not freely and deeply consider your sexual concerns, then find another physician— at least for the sexual part of your health.

On the other hand, do not expect your physician to provide all of the expert diagnoses and treatments that you may need to fully optimize every component of the orgasm system. Best for you would be to put together your own dream team to care for your health and for your sexual health.

When the doctor avoids discussing sex, then the man or woman can be left seeking answers from the internet, the cashier at the sex-toy store, or from a friend. When your team is not diverse, you may experience a physician trying to treat with drugs when you may best be treated with sexual or marriage counseling. Or you may suffer with a physical pain with sex that a trained physician could resolve but not find relief if your only healer is a sex educator who tries to resolve a treatable physical problem with only psychological counseling.

In reality, almost everyone is helped by both physical and psychological healing. For example, even if physical healing improves the desire and orgasmic function of a woman, changing her desire could change the dynamics of her marriage such that her partner now feels threatened or overwhelmed or unable to keep up. So in this case, the improvement of the physical problem with physical therapies could still necessitate marriage or psychological counseling.

Conversely, should a man or woman undergo marriage or sexual counseling and improve desire, then he or she could find that the new demands on the body may reveal the need for physical therapies.

So most people benefit from both physical and psychological therapies. Your best chance for a fully bloomed Garden of Orgasm and Sexual Wellness becomes possible by understanding the components of the orgasm system and putting together a team that addresses all of those components.

I hope you find ways to improve your journey by the information found in this book.

Chapter 1:
Daily Routines to Improve Sex by Dr. Jean Luc Le Provost

Can I help you become happier, healthier, and make positive changes in your life? Is it accurate to say that it can be tough to find your motivation to get there? What drives you? In the past, what emotions have driven you to act differently?

Ultimately, I believe that you want to change. You want to be healthier. You want to conquer your current medical problem, or, if everything is fine, you want to be "better than okay." It's easy to ignore those warning signs of minor health problems as long as those external signs still validate your manhood—strength or sexual performance. As long as you're strong, you're not willing to open up that window.

Everyone, including you and me, respond better to pain instead of pleasure. As long as you look good, you're in a sexually active relationship, and your body works "well enough"— there's no motivation to fix your health. If your sex life is on the decline, you're motivated to have a discussion with me about getting your penis back into prime condition, and we can talk about the lifestyle changes you can make to improve every aspect of your health and longevity. **Sexual wellness is your path to improve your overall health.**

I want to develop trust and rapport with you, with the ultimate goal to balance your entire mind and body— it's all connected. Many physicians are specialists: lung specialists, cardiac specialists, hormone specialists... trained to fix one problem: repair your hand, foot, penis... and ignore the rest. They ignore your other interconnected aspects.

Many physicians run financially incentivized medical businesses, instead of medical practices. They're all about turnover, treating you quickly. If you have erection problems, they want to inject your penis with Trimix. Guaranteed erection. Problem solved in just a few minutes.

That troubles me. As a medical provider, I'm supposed to take care of your entire system. If you have a high risk of cardiovascular disease, heart attack, prostate cancer, obesity, depression, or suicide... I want to do more than simply fix your penis. Those other health problems could manifest themselves in larger forms later.

Heart disease is the number one killer, but my "patient" doesn't want to talk about it. He wants to go back to work, socialize during happy hour, and have sex. Your desire for better sexual health is my opportunity to create a solid relationship with you based on rapport and trust, so we can work on your heart health, energy, diet, digestion, sleep, and other habits. We can treat more than the symptom, we can get to the root cause of many of your problems.

Your Health Snapshot

Let's start with energy. How much energy do you have? More specifically, how long can you walk up stairs? The energy required to walk up stairs equals the amount of energy required for vigorous sex; so, the answer to that question about your endurance walking up stairs tells you about how long a man can last in bed. That realization motivates many men to get back in shape and become aerobically fit.

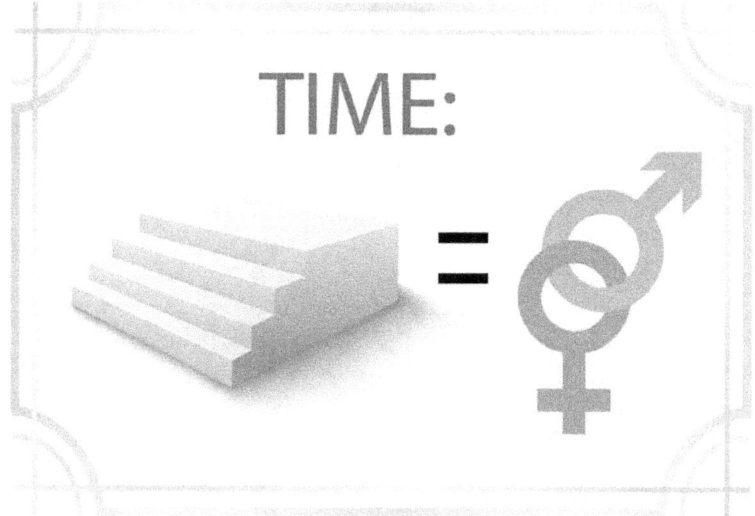

Sexual stamina is about equal to stair stamina.

Are you having problems with your erections? More specifically, how are your morning erections? When you sleep at night, you should have two to five nocturnal erections.

Are you waking up with morning erections more frequently than not? If you don't wake up with an erection four to five times a week, you're more than likely struggling with erection problems. Erections should be a natural part of life. When you sleep and you become erect, that erection is exercise for your penis.

If your penis does not get this "exercise" every morning, or two to three times per night, that's a good indication your overall heart and cardiovascular system is not doing well. Use that as one of your first signs.

Then, if the morning erections do not occur, then ask yourself, "Do I suffer from problems with stress, hormones, or blood flow?"

Blood flow in your penis is similar to the blood flow in your heart. Your penis and heart are closely related. If you have health problems, you see it in your sexual function. If you don't have morning erections, be concerned, look into it, and think about your heart.

Daily Routines

Work out in the morning. Keep it simple.

First, drink a glass of water with a pinch of sea salt for electrolytes, and add a squeeze of lemon. The citrus in the lemon stimulates your liver, opens your detoxification pathways, and hydrates you. Have one big glass of water.

Then, go for a walk 20 to 30 minutes in the morning. That's easy to do.

Set a timer on your phone or watch for 15 minutes. Put your tennis shoes on and walk out the door. It doesn't matter where you go. Walk. Go outside and breathe fresh air. Walk into the morning sunrise, and wake up your body. That morning walk gets your blood moving, wakes you up and is better than any cup of coffee you ever had.

Walking will exercise your heart, stimulate your metabolism, and start the fat-burning process. As soon as your 15-minute timer ends, turn around and head back home.

Do that every morning as part of your routine. When you get back home, then, if you want, drink a cup of coffee or tea.

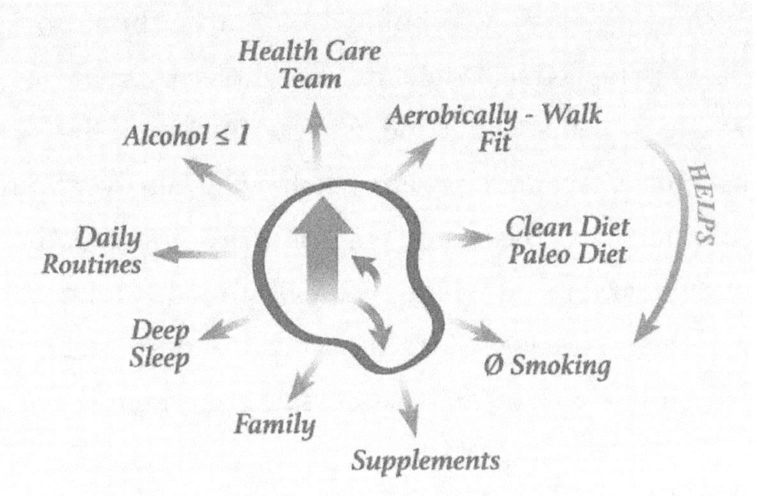

Daily practices that improve sex.

I recommend intermittent fasting by skipping breakfast. Have your cup of coffee, but don't add sugar or creamer. Drink black coffee or green tea.

Then, do your work, and eat lunch around 11AM. Think about the food you put in your body. Take a look at where you're at. Where is your weight and what level of energy do you have?

What you put in your body affects how you feel. It's a hassle to change your diet. First, admit that what you put in your body makes a difference in how you feel.

Second, what can you put in your body? Think from a paleo perspective. Whole foods, whole vegetables, whole proteins, whole meats. You don't need to become a caveman by eating half a chicken every day. Just start with the basics: eliminate processed food and sugar and eat whole foods. Best foods for good health and great sex include avocados, nuts, seeds, almonds, lunch meat, cheeses, salads, protein shakes.

Get creative. That's where meal planning helps.

Start by **eliminating one** thing: sodas. You might be drinking a Diet Coke every day as part of your routine. You open it, it tastes good, and it's fizzy. It brings comfort. Let that go. Soda contains many preservatives, affecting your pancreas and digestion process. It keeps weight on you. Substitute a glass filled halfway with unsweetened juice and one half with your favorite sparkling water.

Add an avocado or an apple to your lunch. Include fattier whole foods, such as nuts and avocados, to keep you feeling more satiated. If you only eat near zero fat foods like apples and salads, you will feel starved and go crazy a few hours after eating. Then, you may revert back to unhealthy eating habits.

Next, **add protein shakes** and other foods from paleo cookbooks. If you make these eating practices something you do for a day or two, then the improvements in sex may be minimal. Instead, for the rest of your life, determine to put good food in your body and to enjoy great sex.

For daily **supplements** to help with erections, take the following: (1) magnesium, (2) vitamin D, (3) B-vitamins. Also, take a good quality cod liver oil—one tablespoon per day. I also recommend zinc.

Zinc is shown to help increase testosterone levels, produce more semen and sperm. Increasing your zinc level will help. Magnesium is also a commonly depleted nutrient in the body.

Make sure you take a good quality zinc supplement. Start with 30 to 90 milligrams of zinc a day with lunch or dinner. It is possible to take so much zinc that it strips your body of copper, but that happens rarely.

Nitric Oxide: The Chief Erection Booster

Many heart medications, erection medications, and supplements mentioned improve nitric oxide, which is what your body uses to make your blood vessels bigger. When your blood vessels get bigger then your penis gets bigger.

Drugs like Viagra and Cialis stimulate this nitric oxide process along with your testosterone activity. When you eat green vegetables, that also stimulates your body to make more nitric oxide. When you walk in the morning, you send a signal to your body that it wants to make more nitric oxide. You tell your heart and penis, "I want more blood flow." When you eat green vegetables, you're telling your heart and your penis, "I want more nitric oxide."

With just a morning walk and eating green vegetables for lunch, you've already done two things today to help you enjoy better sex.

In the evening, come home from work and eat dinner early. Don't go to bed with a full stomach. Keep your diet paleo-leaning: proteins, vegetables, and green vegetables. Eat proteins and plenty of home-cooked whole foods.

Then, just relax. Let go of the stress created during the day. Your mental health is important. Reduce your stress to reduce your risk of heart disease. Take your body out of sympathetic stimulation (fight-or-flight mode) and towards parasympathetic (relaxed) mode. Sex and erections like parasympathetic. Your wife, your kids, and you personally, all of you, just relax. Take your spouse on a 20 to 30-minute relaxing evening stroll. Give your food time to digest. You will sleep better.

Sleep Habits to Improve Your Health

You most likely don't get enough sleep. You go to bed too late and wake up too early, or perhaps you don't get enough deep sleep. Try to go to bed with very little food in your stomach, in a parasympathetic, relaxed mode.

If you prefer supplements to help you sleep, 5-HTP is one of my favorite supplements. It is made from the tryptophan protein. It converts to melatonin or serotonin in your brain to provide a deeper sleep. It is not a drug, will not knock you out, and does not make you drowsy. It helps you get a deeper sleep.

5-HTP produces more serotonin and melatonin in your brain, which helps you sleep better. You can have the perfect diet and a personal trainer, but if you don't get sleep, you age faster. You have an increased risk of heart disease, wrinkles on your face, grumpiness, and increased weight.

When you sleep, your body resets and recharges. Your body produces melatonin, which also fights cancer. With deep sleep, your serotonin (the happiness hormone) levels are better when you wake up. Your muscles and brain repair themselves. **Do not short change yourself on sleep.**

Optionally, you can take melatonin combined with 5-HTP. When you buy melatonin products, look at the label. It should say "micronized lipid matrix melatonin." A micronized lipid matrix is a small molecule which ensures its absorption into your body. Many melatonin supplements on the market are cheap and not a micronized lipid matrix. Without the lipid matrix, melatonin will not absorb into your body.

Anytime you try something "natural" and it "doesn't work"— examine the quality of that natural product. Then, ask, "Did I take enough of it?"

For example, oftentimes, doctors recommend 1 mg melatonin at bedtime. But, you can take more than that: 5, 10, 20, or even 30 milligrams at night. Some cancer patients take 60 to 100 milligrams of melatonin per day.

If you want to try melatonin to improve your sleep, start with 3 to 5 milligrams 30 minutes before bed, and add 5-HTP. Then, go to bed on time. Shut down your computer, TV, and phone one hour before bed. Tell your body and your family to get ready for bed.

Again, if you wake in the night, or when you wake in the morning, notice your erections. Do you have erections during the night? Are you waking up with a morning erection?

The size of your penis shrinks with fewer erections. Erections are an indication of your heart AND sexual health. Nobody wants a smaller penis, but that's one of the concerns I hear from my older patients. "I feel my penis is smaller." You use it or lose it.

If you don't get nocturnal erections, you don't get blood flow and exercise for your penis. If you don't get that exercise, tissue decreases in size— in this case, your penis! We all think, "If my penis isn't getting exercise, that means my heart is not getting exercise."

Stop This Sex Killer

Your sexual health is affected by smoking and alcohol. Men often think those two things things act as a social lubricant with the bar scene and with sex. If alcohol is a consistent part of your life, you won't be eating well, exercising well, or sleeping well. Now, most experts consider more than one alcoholic drink per day to be too much.

Smoking, of course, affects your lungs, increases your risk of cancer, and adds toxins to your system, that your body spends energy fighting. But, smoking also causes inflammation in your blood vessels including your penis and eventually leads to erectile dysfunction. Since smoking only causes harm, everyone on some level eventually knows that quitting would be best, but since quitting smoking can be so difficult, I'll offer a few tips to help you be successful.

First, you must WANT to quit smoking. Be honest with yourself. Until you really want to quit, you won't.

Second, have a purpose for quitting other than your health. What is more important to you than cigarettes? Not something superficial like saving money for your car, truck, or house. Look inside your heart and ask, "What's important to me?" The answer to this question must be more important than cigarettes. Usually, it comes back to a child, your lover, or something else that's greater to you than even your health. Now, tie quitting to your being there in a more meaningful way for that person or cause.

Third, don't be afraid to ask for assistance: prescriptions, nicotine gum, counseling, quit smoking programs, and acupuncture. All of these interventions can help you quit— do them all at the same time.

Look into your heart. You are a human being. Connect with yourself and your emotions. Quit smoking and enjoy great sex.

Summary

When you enjoy these small habit changes and successes, you become happier and feel better. Your biggest challenge is on the mental side. Create a new habit. Make the decision in your life that you are in control of these choices. That is your biggest challenge.

You can do it. You might feel resistance. Change "small" habits like soda. Don't cheat yourself of two hours of sleep a night. Don't drink too much coffee. Be careful about having that one Snack Pack every day at lunch. Over the course of time, those types of habits have led you to a tired, overweight, and unhappy situation. You will feel your life on the decline.

Consider a wake-up routine that includes water and a walk. Practice a paleo morning breakfast, light lunch, and dinner. Leave out diet drinks. Relax, get to bed at a decent time, regularly, and get a good rest.

Your body and mind are connected — you hear a loud noise behind you and your heart rate increases. Your brain is attached to your pituitary glands, which is attached to your other glands, affecting your hormones and then your cells. It's not simply a spiritual relationship. These are mechanical, physiological medical processes.

If you have been experiencing sexual health problems like erectile dysfunction, or sex is not good as it used to be, be honest with yourself. Don't be afraid to seek help. This is your start to a better high-quality life. Not just more pleasure, but deeper relationships, confidence, and happiness.

It takes courage to look deep down and understand your emotions. Be open to the possibility of connecting with yourself to balance that mind-body relationship. You need this. You have built a defensive emotional wall that has protected you from harm, but it has also stifled your growth. You are in a safe place to not only find hope in your present situation, but get excited about your own possibilities for the future.

Steps to Your Sexual Wellness

1. Thoughtfully create a definite daily routine that improves cardiac and sexual health. You don't need expensive equipment to stay fit. Go for a short walk or run. Involve your spouse and kids on your journey to a healthy lifestyle.
2. Strategically choose what food you put inside your body. Your diet is a huge part of improving your health. The food that you put in your body affects how you feel. Cut out soda and sugar. Practice intermittent fasting.
3. Supplement your diet with zinc, magnesium, B-vitamins, C, and nitric oxide.
4. Improve your sleeping habits.
5. Stop smoking. What could be a few good reasons to quit?

More About Dr. Jean Luc Le Provost

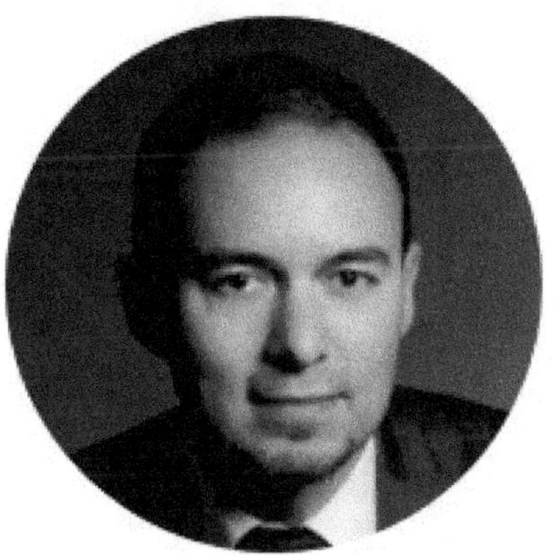

Dr. Jean Luc Le Provost's extensive background in nutrition, personal training, pharmaceuticals, and alternative medical therapies provides his patients with the most up-to-date knowledge in the world of integrative medicine.

His goal is to improve your quality of life and help you live your life to its fullest potential.

- **Website:** PhoenixMensHealthCenter.com
- **Location:** Phoenix, Arizona, USA
- **Phone Number:** 602-908-5422

48

Chapter 2:
Sleep, Sex & You
(No Sleep, No Sex)
by Dr. Prabhat Soni

It is true that there is no sexual wellness if you have no good sleep. Sex is an important part of life. Even a transient sexual thought can give you positive energy to improve your sleep and feeling of wellbeing.

Despite multiple factors affecting sexual wellness and a multi-modality approach is the right way to address each issue, sleep is the biggest and primary issue to be fixed first to enjoy the fullness of life. Using a pill to fix sexual need is like putting a band-aid for immediate gain without paying attention to the underlying problems.

Today we are facing a medical tsunami (better called a sexual tsunami) because of a rapidly growing problem worldwide of Obesity and its multiple complications specially affecting Sleep disorders (sleep deprivation, sleep apnea, insomnia) and much more including hormones. These issues affect not only our overall health but also our sexual wellness.

"It's getting late. How about if we get it together tomorrow?"

"I think about sex a lot, but I lack the energy to enjoy it."

"I'm too tired for sex this evening."

Have you made such comments or felt the sentiment behind them? More than likely you have.

Science & the Importance of Sleep

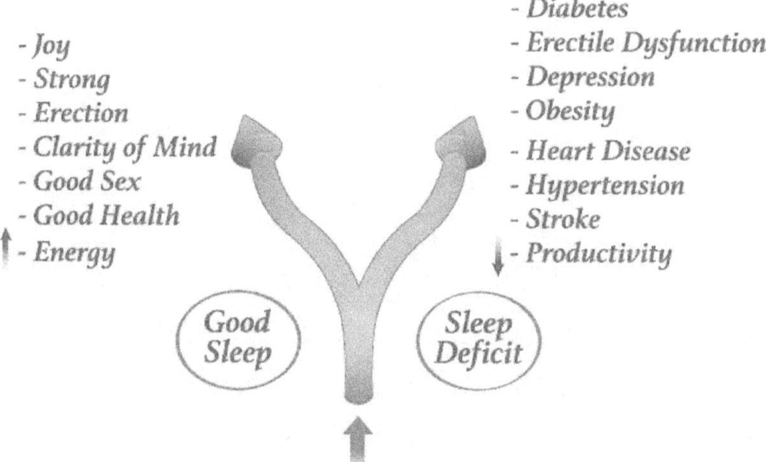

Why to choose good sleep.

As a medical doctor, I work with patients who express a variety of concerns about their health. Often, at some point, the topic of sexual wellness arises. Many sexually unsatisfied patients tell me that they feel tired or fatigued even before sex— and sometimes fall asleep while in the act of sexual intercourse!

Good sexual health is the result of physical, mental and spiritual factors that are in balance with each other. Because our sexuality is so basic to who we are as human beings, any problem with sexual wellness should not be ignored.

The more I've worked with patients, the more I've come to realize that there is a critical connection between sex and sleep. Basically, there is no sexual wellness without good sleep!

I cannot overemphasize this important point enough: *Sleep is the most important vital sign of our well-being and sexual wellness.*

Many men and women experience one or more of the following states mentioned below, when it comes to the connection between sex and sleep. Do you identify with any of the following?

- *No sleep* means no sex.
- *Too much sleep* means that you should wake up to get a check-up to rule out narcolepsy or some other condition.
- *Too little sleep* (being sleep deprived in quantity or quality) means that you wake up feeling tired and fatigued. More than likely, you also are experiencing poor libido.
- The worst part of no sleep is that people sleep for ever because of complications of sleep deprivation or NO SLEEP.

Interestingly, whether you are rich or poor, you want three things in life: to look good, to feel great, and to perform well in your daily activities. Achieving these three things is just the beginning. Remember that the ultimate goal is to achieve a greater sense of satisfaction in your life— physically, mentally, spiritually and sexually.

But what stands in the way of achieving these goals could be poor quality sleep, which affects everything you do and can drastically impact your state of sexual wellness.

Okay, sleep is important. "But why?"— you might be asking. Let's take a closer look at the topic of sleep itself.

First of all, sleep is a necessary and recurring state of the body and the mind— one in which the body's systems are in an anabolic state that helps to rejuvenate the nervous, skeletal, immune, and muscular systems. These systems are vital in the maintenance of your body's essential functions.

Sleep is divided into four stages. There are two basic types of sleep stages: non-Rapid Eye Movement (non-REM) and Rapid Eye Movement (REM) sleep. During the three non-REM stages, your brain does not use as much energy. During the REM stage, according to the Sleep Foundation: "Brain activity picks up, nearing levels seen when you're awake..." and "the body experiences atonia, which is a temporary paralysis of the muscles," except for "the eyes and the muscles that control breathing."[1]

During these sleep stages, there is a 44% reduction in the cerebral metabolic rate for glucose. Sleep provides your mind and body with a power boost and gives you a fresh start for your daily life.

What happens when you don't get enough sleep? You become a sleep debtor!

Sleep debt is like having a credit card or mortgage. You are born with a "sleep loan." Every day, you work a full day, then pay back seven to eight hours of sleep to keep that sleep debt current. Unfortunately, in these "modern" times, the debt is not paid back. Whenever we need more time, we cut our sleep hours and accumulate more sleep debt.

If you fall too far behind in paying a home mortgage, the bank eventually takes your home. Did you know that a similar thing happens when your sleep debt is too high? Except that the "home" you lose is your living body!

To continue with this analogy, a bank sends warning letters before they take your home. Similarly, your sleep bank provides *"warning letters"* in the form of:

- hypertension
- diabetes
- weight gain
- snoring
- sleep apnea
- heart attack

- stroke
- low libido
- erectile dysfunction
- lack of concentration / memory impairment

Facing the Truth About Sleep Disorders

Unfortunately, 50- to 70-million Americans suffer from sleep disorders.[2] Chances are, you are one of them.

In fact, 30% of the U.S. population has reported sleep disturbances lasting several nights per month, and about 10% of the US population suffer from a clinically significant sleep disorder.[3]

What is a sleep disorder? A sleep disorder could refer to parasomnia, insomnia, circadian rhythm disorders, sleep-related breathing disorders, sleep-related movement disorders, central disorders of hypersomnolence, and so forth.

Probably the most common sleep disorder is insomnia, which receives the most public attention.[4]

It is both a disorder and a symptom that is characterized by chronic dissatisfaction with sleep quantity or quality. It is associated with difficulty falling asleep, frequent night-time awakenings, difficulty returning to sleep, and possibly awakening earlier in the morning than you desire.[5]

Sleep disorders get substantial attention because of their high prevalence rates and negative health outcomes. Before electricity was invented, people had no choice but to sleep at night. There was no television or cell phone to cut into night-time sleep hours.

These days, many of us, whenever we need more time in our daily life, cut our sleep hours and end up in serious sleep problems, which interfere with sexual wellness.

Common Problems
Affecting Sleep & Sex

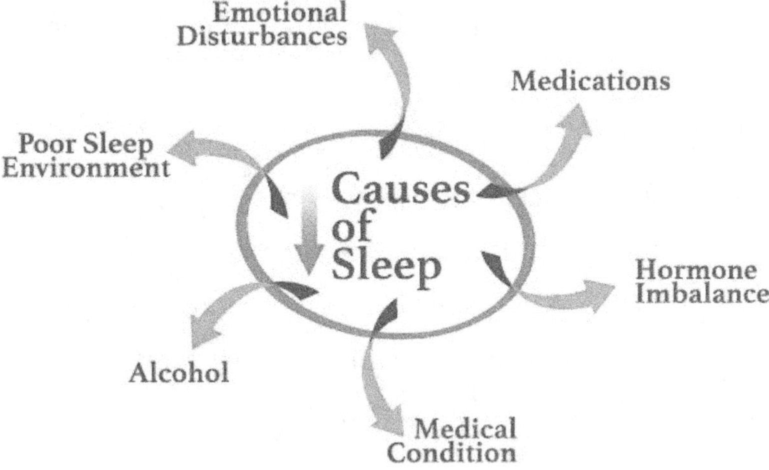

Enemies of healthful sleep.

As we outlined in the earlier list, the impact of sleep indebtedness is huge. Here we will focus on a number of the negative conditions that can arise from, and contribute to, sleep deprivation.

Obesity

Whether we want to admit it or not, we are facing a medical tsunami in the form of the rapidly growing, worldwide problem of obesity, or excessive weight gain.

Obesity has been linked to sleep disorders, including sleep deprivation, sleep apnea, and insomnia. It is ironic that while sleep deprivation can lead to obesity, obesity can lead to sleep deprivation and sleep apnea!

Sleep Apnea

As the obesity rate has increased around the world, sleep apnea has become more of a problem. Obstructive Sleep Apnea can be a drag on your love life, taking the form of erectile dysfunction (ED) in men, and loss of libido in women.

A clear link has been made between OSA and issues associated with sexual functioning. For example, when researchers studied male patients with Obstructive Sleep Apnea (OSA), they noticed a high incidence of Erectile Dysfunction (ED) and low serum testosterone levels. There is also a link between anti-depressants and stimulant medications used for narcolepsy and ED, but the majority of research has been done on OSA.

In male patients tested for suspected OSA, 69% with OSA also had ED. Only 34% of patients without OSA suffered from ED. This study seems to establish a link between sleep deprivation and sexual performance.

There was a significant improvement in sleep apnea after CPAP use, but no significant increase in testosterone levels. CPAP did not impact psychological, hormonal, or biochemical profiles. Still, multiple studies have found that there is a significant increase in erectile function and overall satisfaction (including sexual satisfaction) after CPAP treatment. The sexual-function success rate was 24.8% with CPAP alone and 61.1% in combination with an erectile dysfunction medication like Viagra.

Many studies show that ***combination therapies may be the best approach to treat both sleep apnea and ED***. While the majority of research has been done on male patients, similar findings have been found in female patients as well. OSA is more common in men than in women, but the disorder has similar effects on both genders: impairing sexual function and lowering sex hormones.

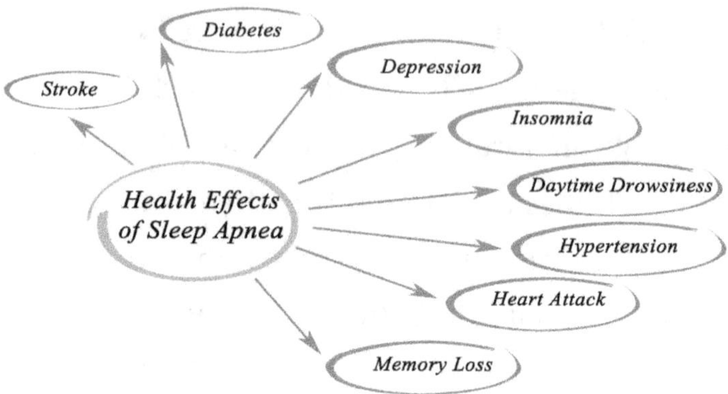

Basically, poor circulation is the root cause of erectile dysfunction and other sexual dysfunction. The most common causes of poor circulation are hypertension, diabetes, and medication side effects.

Depression

Unfortunately, medications used to treat depression often have a negative effect on sex that could lead to sexual dysfunction. With antidepressants like Zoloft, Paxil, SSRIs, or similar medications, a person typically experiences almost no REM sleep. For men, that might mean no morning erection, while for women, it could mean low libido or vaginal dryness or both.

Hypertension

High blood pressure is a common cause of ED linked to poor circulation. Medications like diuretics slow down blood flow and deplete serum levels of zinc, which help the testosterone-making process. Beta-blockers (such as metoprolol and atenolol) help lower blood pressure by blocking certain receptors in our nervous system, but they interfere with the part of the male nervous system responsible for erections.

Diabetes

Sleep indebtedness could lead to diabetes, which, in turn, promotes obesity, sleep apnea, low libido, and hormone imbalance. Erection dysfunction is affected by insufficient blood flow due to microvascular disease and neuropathy. Low testosterone levels (which affect erections) are found in about 25% of diabetic patients.

Chronic Stress and Adrenal Fatigue

Stress affects your sex life in many ways. In men, high cortisol suppresses testosterone. Over time, a man's adrenal glands become unable to make more cortisol, and most patients end up with adrenal fatigue.

Stress affects post-menopausal women especially when their thyroid, progesterone and testosterone hormones are also low, but stress is no respecter of persons, impacting everyone regardless of gender and age.

At this point, you could be thinking that poor quality sleep wreaks havoc on the human body, and you would be correct! The interconnection between sleep and sex is unmistakable!

Here's a handy summary of common factors affecting sleep and sexual wellness:

1. **Medications.** Antidepressants, anti-hypertensives, and sedatives.
2. **Poor sleep hygiene.** Good sleep hygiene involves limiting daytime naps, avoiding stimulants (nicotine) close to bedtime, avoiding foods that interfere with sleep, establishing a bedtime routine, making sure the bedroom is comfortable, non-stimulating, and conducive to sleep.
3. **Hormonal imbalance.** Your testosterone and cortisol levels could be out of balance. This is often a problem in post-menopausal females.

4. **Medical conditions.** Hypertension and diabetes could be playing a role in sleep and sex at the same time.

5. **Alcohol and substance-use disorders.** Alcohol consumption close to bedtime. Use of illegal substances, especially stimulants.

6. **Individual circumstance.** Having a sex partner who has a sleep disturbance can affect the quality of life for both of you.

So, now the question remains: "How do I avoid or overcome the problems of sleep deprivation and sexual dysfunction?" The following section provides some helpful guidelines and suggestions to maximize your sleep quotient and enhance your enjoyment of one of life's greatest gifts: the gift of sexuality.

Solutions to Improve Sleep and Sex

After knowing the importance of sleep and the problems caused by poor sleep, what can you do? How can you get good sleep and increase sexual wellness at the same time?

Tip #1: Medication is not the solution to every problem. Minimize your use of medications when possible.

Tip #2: Discipline yourself. Stay natural and romantic. Treat your partner the way you want to be treated. Be happy. Make people around you happy as well.

Tip #3: Practice *sleep hygiene*. Use your bedroom only for sleep and sex.

Tip #4: With sleep disorders, if your partner is snoring at night and you are both not getting restful sleep, seek medical attention for your partner. Consult a sleep Doctor. Order a sleep study to determine if your partner can benefit from a CPAP mask or oral appliance.

Tip #5: Remember that obesity and sleep apnea go together. A sleep apnea patient should use a CPAP machine as well as seriously lose weight.

Tip #6: To *improve circulation* to the sex organs, you could consider a combination of treatments including:

- **Platelet-Rich Plasma:** P-Shot® for males and O-Shot® for females. (A breakthrough treatment invented by Dr. Charles Runels to help the problem of sexual wellness).

- **Stem cells:** to grow new arteries. These can be taken from adipose tissue, bone marrow, umbilical cord, amniotic fluid, or exosomes.
- **Shock wave therapy:** specifically, extracorporeal shock waves break up plaque formation in blood vessels and stimulate the growth of new blood vessels in your penis or genitalia. This improves sexual function in men and women.

Tip #7: If you suffer from hypertension and/or diabetes: ask your doctor to modify your medications so they don't affect your sexual function and weight gain. Alpha blockers (like Norvasc) and ACEI (lisinopril) are good choices for blood pressure control. Metformin is a good choice for diabetes.

Tip #8: In the cases of insomnia and depression, these are frequently treated with Ambien and Zoloft. Ask your doctor if these medications could be modified to keep your REM sleep intact and avoid weight gain. My go-to choices are melatonin and 5-HTP for insomnia, and Wellbutrin for depression.

Tip #9: Check how you look, especially the "look" of your entire body, and not only your face. Many physicians offer options including botox, fillers, or PDO thread lifts. Imagine how your look will change if you combine any of these with medical weight loss or body sculpting. Even just losing weight and exercising could make a big difference too!

Tip #10: Take note of your energy level. If you feel tired or fatigued, you might turn off your partner even if you look extremely beautiful or handsome. Have your hormones, especially thyroid, cortisol and testosterone, checked. Your hormones must be balanced to help you feel energetic.

Tip #11: Learn how to remain calm and to stay in the present moment. Don't be embarrassed if you find yourself in need of extra help. There's no shame in a man boosting his sexual performance by adding an ED medication (like Viagra) with testosterone. In some cases, a bi-mix and tri-mix injection fifteen minutes before sexual intercourse could help him.

Conclusion

Your blood pressure, heart rate, and breathing rate are all vital signs. But your sleep is another important vital sign, and many medical clinics ignore this factor. You need good sleep for good health, which means physical health, mental health and a great quality of life.

Consider that you need good sleep to help boost your immunity and balance your hormones so that you can better win fights against many diseases, including COVID-19.

Pay attention to early warning signs. For men, having poor or no erection on awakening is not a good sign. For men and women, feeling tired when you wake up or needing a nap during daytime could be indirect evidence of poor sleep. Don't wait. Instead, take immediate action, and contact a sleep specialist to rule out any sleep disorder.

Quantity is a requirement but Quality of sleep is important as well (insufficient sleep, disturbed sleep, sleep deprivation and many other sleep disorders, including sleep apnea) to affect many aspects of your health including sexual function.

Regenerative medicine has revolutionized sexual medicine treatment with Platelet-Rich Plasma. P-Shot®, O- Shot®, stem cells, and shock wave therapy combined with hormone balance (testosterone pellets). These are life-changing modalities that you should consider, if appropriate for your situation.

Erectile dysfunction or any sexual dysfunction could be a consequence of several sleep disorders. If this is a problem or is developing into a problem for you, please get a referral to a sleep medicine specialist. Sleep doctor will order a home sleep testing (HST) or in-lab sleep test (PSG) according to your needs and fix the underlying sleep issue.

In this chapter, we have taken a short journey into many of the problems and solutions related to sleep and sex. I hope you have come to the conclusion that sexual wellness cannot be achieved without good quality sleep. May you enjoy both now and always!

More About Dr. Prabhat Soni

Dr. Prabhat Soni is an American MD board-certified in eight specialties, including internal medicine, pulmonary, critical care, sleep, obesity, aesthetic anti-aging, and regenerative medicine. Dr. Soni was recently featured on Fox

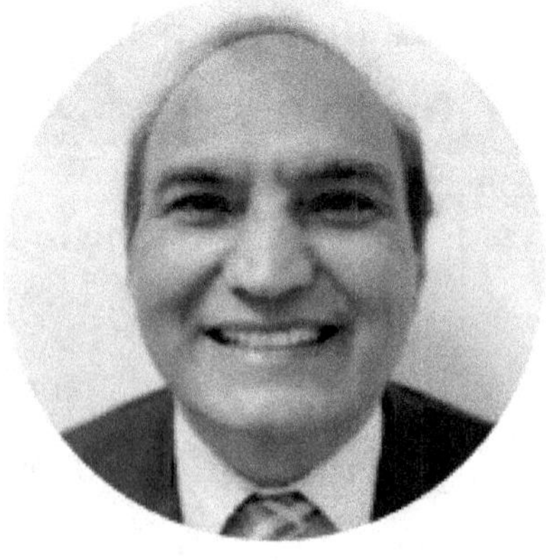

News-31 Colorado for his stem-cell miracle on behalf of a critically ill patient dying from Covid-19, but saved through stem-cell therapy that was FDA-approved for emergency compassionate use.

- Prabhat Soni MD, DABSM (sleep), ABAARM (stem cell)
- Medical Director, GIOSTAR (stem cell)
- 2519 Ave O, Brooklyn, NY 11210
- 718-787-1900 office, 917-803-4136 cell
- SoniMedical.com
- prabhatsoni106@gmail.com

References

1. National Heart, Lung and Blood Institute, 2003 National Sleep Disorders Research Plan, National Center on Sleep Disorders Research; U.S. Department of Health and Human Services, National Institutes of Health, National Heart, Lung, and Blood Institute, National Center on Sleep Disorders Research, Trans-NIH Sleep Research Coordinating Committee; Jan 2003.

2. Suni, E., "Stages of Sleep," SleepFoundation.org, 2019 Aug.

3. Ram, S., et.al, "Prevalence and impact of sleep disorders and sleep habits in the United States," Sleep Breath, 2010 Feb;14(1):63-70.

4. Basta, M., et.al., "Chronic Insomnia and Stress," Sleep Med Clin, 2007 June; 2(2): 279-291.

5. American Academy of Sleep Medicine, International Classification of Sleep Disorders, 3rd ed. (Darien, IL USA, 2014.

6. Sullivan, C.E., et.al., "Reversal of Obstructive Sleep Apnea by Continuous Positive Airway Pressure Applied Through the Nose"; The Lancet, 1(8225): 862-5; May 1981.

Chapter 3:
Regenerative Therapy
for Enhanced Sexual Wellness
by Dr. Cristyn Watkins

We can improve the health and function of the genitalia by using a variety of strategies to *improve tissue health at the cellular level.*

The most common method to improve tissue health is *hormonal therapies*. Hormones act as chemical messengers that tell the cell to improve protein synthesis and cellular function. We can also use the newest strategies to improve the tissue of the genitalia at the cellular level. These therapies include peptides, platelet-rich plasma, ozone, exosomes, amnion, and topical cell modulators like CBD and vasodilators.

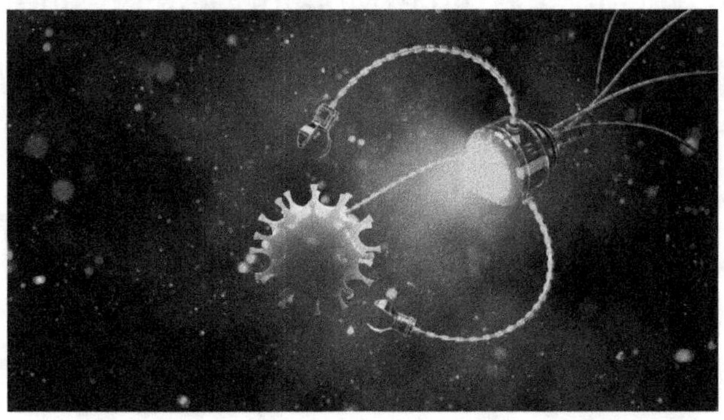

All of these cellular therapies work together to promote growth in healthy tissue, activate messenger protein signaling to the area of concern, and improve tissues to function more youthfully.

How My Personal Health Battles Taught Me a Better Way

I have a special interest in autoimmune disorders, chronic inflammation and regenerative therapies due to my own health battles. When I was 12, I caught a cold but seemed to be much more sick than expected. It was not improving and after several weeks, we realized it was mono and I was hospitalized for six weeks. The doctors monitored my blood count and liver enzymes, but the situation continued to worsen. Eventually, I had jaundice and severe abdominal pain and they still couldn't figure out what was going on.

Finally, the doctors did exploratory surgery and removed my spleen (3 of them!) and my gallbladder (with 9 gallstones!) and realized something more serious was the culprit.

They were eventually able to understand it was due to a hereditary blood disorder called spherocytosis. I was the first female in my family to have it.

After I had my spleen removed, I thought, "There must be a better way to help people with immune and chronic disease."

Over the years, my immune system worsened. When I became sick, recovery time would take twice as long as everyone else and I would miss school and activities for prolonged periods. I knew there had to be a better answer than medications and "time."

I decided that I wanted to become a physician and that I wanted to focus on wellness— not just "treat" the disease and symptoms, but rather treat and fix the cause. Traditional medicine is great at acute care and at prescribing medications, but it's not as helpful at fixing the root cause of chronic disease and a compromised immune system. So, after eight years of private practice as a Family Physician, I decided that I needed to do something more to help people who suffer from the ravages of autoimmune disease, problems like chronic pain, fatigue, headaches, and the sexual dysfunctions that come from hormone disorders and inflammation.

At the time I started practicing functional medicine five years ago (and obtaining my 2nd board certification in the specialty), I suffered with pain, fatigue, headaches, and anxiety. I also had unexplained infertility and had to conceive all of my four children through in vitro fertilization. Obviously, something was off but my traditional physicians could not find any reason other than "stress." I knew there was something wrong, but no doctor could diagnose my problems as my lab results were all "perfect."

I started to look for causes myself with my new training and eventually discovered that I have low progesterone, estrogen dominance, Lyme disease, chronic mold with yeast, and extremely high toxins in my system.

I realized that during medical school is when the anxiety and migraines first began. Then after I lost my first child eight years ago is when the chronic muscle pain and fatigue started. It was debilitating. I followed functional nutrition guidelines. I went gluten-free and followed an anti-inflammatory diet. I started supplements to increase nutrients and to assist with detox. That helped, but only 60 to 70 percent. I knew there was a way I could feel 90 percent better.

I started to explore and research Regenerative Medicine and began further training. In the past I had taken Cymbalta, pain meds, anti-inflammatories, and muscle relaxers for fibromyalgia pain with little results. But, then after using what I had learned in functional and regenerative medicine and trying exosomes, PRP and ozone, my pain was completely gone in four days. Since intravenous ozone helps treat fungal disease, Lyme disease, bacterial infections, and viral infections, I implemented ozone for 10 weeks. I also received IV exosomes, the O-Shot® procedure, and Ozone/PRP trigger point injections. I have personally experienced every procedure that I perform in my Aesthetic, Regenerative and Wellness practice.

As a result, my cognitive function returned and I live with drastically less chronic pain and fatigue and my sex life became amazing.

Because I overcame these medical issues, and learned how to help others with similar problems, I expanded my medical practice from a two-employee small practice in a 1,500-square foot space into 2 locations with 20 employees and 10,000 square feet of total space. And all this while being a mother to a 7-year-old boy and 4-year-old twin girls.

Let's talk about some of the tools that I used to help change my life and the lives of the people who come to me for help.

Platelet-Rich Plasma (PRP)

Platelet-rich plasma contains growth factors that heal tissue, produce neovascularization (new blood vessels and nerve growth), new collagen, and reduce inflammation.

Making PRP is a very simple process. First, we draw blood into a specialized tube that is approved by the FDA for the preparation of PRP to go back into the body. The tube is then placed into an FDA-approved centrifuge that separates red blood cells from platelets. We then inject the PRP back into the body to improve tissue health in the area where it is needed.

Platelet-Rich Plasma (PRP) acts like a beacon to signal messenger proteins which migrate through the bloodstream to the place where we inject the PRP to heal the tissue. When we inject PRP into the vagina using this specialized technique, it's called the O-Shot® procedure. When we inject it into the penis, we call it the P-Shot® or Priapus Shot® procedure.

I use O-Shot® and P-Shot® to treat incontinence, erectile dysfunction, vaginal dryness, low arousal, and lichen sclerosus.

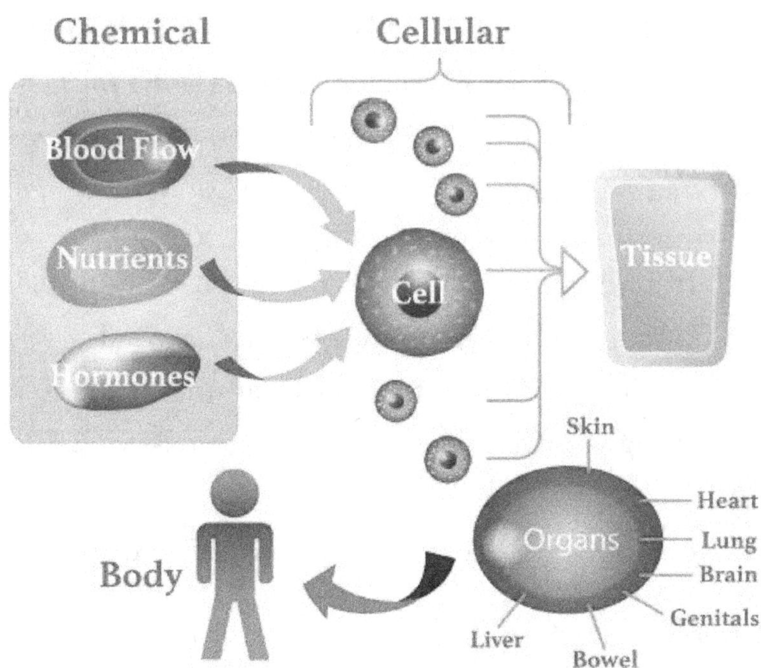

Improving cells improves the entire body.

PRP treatment is also useful for joint pain, muscle injuries, arthritis, trigger points and fibromyalgia pain. Because the injection of PRP causes angiogenesis, tissue repair, new collagen and nerves to grow, athletes have been using PRP for over fifteen years. The strategy is so effective, PRP was banned by the Olympics temporarily as something that gave an unfair advantage. Veterinarians also use PRP to help race horses recover from training and to run faster.

Why should professional athletes and race horses have exclusive use of PRP? We simply use that same healing strategy to help people regenerate the tissue of the genitalia, joints, and muscles and they can live a fully functional life.

I call PRP "Liquid Gold" as it can be used for multiple conditions: pain, autoimmune disorders, sexual rejuvenation, hair restoration, facial aesthetics, body contouring, and almost anything musculoskeletal.

Amazing Sex After Breast Cancer

A female patient visited me a few years ago. She was sobbing as she told me about another physician who had literally torn her vagina, causing bleeding and trauma during a pelvic exam. She had not had sex in many years due to vaginal dryness, pain, and lack of desire following her battle with breast cancer that required radiation, chemotherapy, and a double mastectomy. She felt unattractive, broken, and was worried about divorce.

Her situation affected her relationship with her husband of 40+ years and she was afraid of losing her marriage. She could not attempt to have intercourse with him, as it was painful for her, even with lubricants.

She was 62 and that is simply too young to quit having sex.

We discussed the best options, considering her symptoms: vaginal dryness, pain, lack of desire, and libido. She was post breast cancer treatment, and therefore, her oncologist had told her that hormone therapy was not an option for her.

We designed a ***tailor-made, combination therapy*** of O-Shot® (PRP), exosomes, ThermiVa (radio-frequency), peptides (PT-141), and a compounded topical cream called "Scream Cream." I also put her on a CBD lubricant to heighten arousal and give lubrication while we were waiting for these therapies to begin working.

In addition to the usual O-Shot® procedure, I injected exosomes into the perineum and vulvar areas to accelerate the healing and rejuvenation of the tissue. This concept also applies to injecting a joint, scar or muscle. It increases blood flow, brings oxygen to the area, increases nerve supply, signals tissue healing, produces collagen and remodeling as PRP does.

I saw her only a month later, after her first treatment, for her second ThermiVa appointment and she was bawling.

Crying, she hugged me and said, "I don't think I even need the second and third treatment. My sex life is back! Our marriage is better than ever!" She now has better sex AFTER breast cancer treatment than she did before her cancer.

I completed her ThermiVa series to enhance results as recommended and also put her on compounded peptide PT-141 which helps to increase sexual desire and function1. It works on the hypothalamus and induces rapid onset of arousal. It is FDA approved for women for hypo-arousal and there's an FDA-approved prescription version now. There are two compound pharmacists I trust who make individual-for-each-patient, custom-designed sexual wellness compounds. I can combine compounded PT-141, "scream cream", and nasal oxytocin for a synergistic effect in most women.

I love **oxytocin to get an "afterglow"** (even without having sex if you want). Young patients with a lost libido explain PT-141 (especially combined with oxytocin) is almost like being on "a love drug" when they have sexual intercourse.

Exosomes to Improve the Love Organs

Exosomes are acellular, meaning they are not a cell. They are **proteins that carry messenger RNA from one cell to another** to regenerate the next cell. Instead of it being an actual cell, like stem cells, they are more of a messenger system that signals other cells to regenerate and heal.

Exosomes[4] are extremely small particles, 40 nanometers. They take information from one cell and tell the next cell how to appropriately make new healthier tissue. They're not rejected or perceived as foreign. They influence the growth of the target cells, promote regeneration, and are anti-inflammatory. They are anti-fibrotic, which is important in patients with Peyronie's Disease or for those suffering with vascular conditions that cause erectile dysfunction; exosomes improve endothelial function to create a more firm erection.

Exosomes reduce oxidative stress damage and help improve smooth muscle. There are over 40 growth factors present in mesenchymal or MSC exosomes[5] including TGF beta-3, IL-6, IL-106. They can down-regulate certain unwanted cells and up-regulate other cells to reduce inflammation and cause regeneration of healthy tissue. Think of exosomes as the quarterback, telling the team of cells what to do to generate healthier tissue.

People worry about the word "growth" and tumors. We don't fully know if stem cells that are prepared outside the body and then injected back into the body are tumorigenic or not. We don't believe they are, but we have no proof of that; which is one reason why stem cells are controlled by the FDA. This is not the same as PRP, which simply increases and regenerates the cells and growth factors in your own body in the area of injection; which is one of the reasons that *PRP is NOT regulated by the FDA— it's just your own blood.* The same is true for Exosomes, which are not cells and not regulated by the FDA. Even better, we DO have strong evidence that exosomes up-regulate tumor suppression to help fight cancer and tumor growth.

When I perform the O-Shot® or P-Shot® procedure for my patients, I will often mix the PRP with exosomes for an enhanced version of the procedure— exosomes in the same syringe with PRP. The combination of the two can be amazing for some people with the PRP acting as the scaffolding and "food" for the exosomes and the PRP turning into a platelet-rich fibrin matrix which forms a scaffolding that holds the growth factors in place.

We inject the O-Shot® in the usual places: the clitoris, the periurethral space, and sometimes in the vulva; so, *imagine all of these areas waking up* and you get an idea of what is possible.

Ozone

Ozone is a gas made up of three oxygen atoms (O3). Oxygen (O2) is supplied from an oxygen tank and put through an Ozonator, which adds an extra oxygen molecule. Our bodies make ozone, which binds to hemoglobin in the body, reduces oxidation and free radicals, but also allows us to take in more oxygen and make better use of it. This results in improved circulation and overall bodily functions such as cognition, immunity and other cellular functions.

As we age, there is oxidative stress and increased inflammation. Eventually, this decreases our production of ozone, decreases cellular functions and accelerates the aging process.

Ozone can also destroy bacteria, viruses, fungi, yeast and protozoa, by activating the immune system. I use this for topical wound healing and intravenously to help treat chronic infections such as Lyme, bacteria, viruses, mold, and yeast.

Ozone is drawn from the ozonator with a syringe and "bagged", injected directly into tissues, or intravenously. It is combined with PRP and/or exosomes for enhanced results. PRP and ozone supply the exosomes with immediate scaffolding and nourishment. It's also locally oxygenated, which stimulates and activates the PRP almost immediately.

I inject it out of the syringe as if it were PRP or a liquid, immediately into the area of treatment; the procedure is done like a steroid or PRP injection and is essentially painless.

For intravenous ozone, I start with a one-liter bag of sterile saline and remove some of the fluid from the bag to leave space. We then add your pre-drawn blood, heparin, and ozone into the bag.

By mixing the ozone with the hemoglobin in your blood, we attach that O3 to the hemoglobin and oxygenate it. The more blood we draw and the more ozone we add to that IV bag[7], the more we oxygenate your hemoglobin to be delivered to the rest of your body.

Then we run that mixture slowly (over 30-60 minutes) into your body and you go home feeling great!

Using IV ozone, we treat chronic fatigue, fibromyalgia, Lyme disease, autoimmune disease, heart problems, peripheral neuropathy, asthma, and COPD. I've never had a patient have a side effect from ozone. Most people feel elated, a sense of clarity, and energized. Their pain also decreases and they feel a sense of joy and calm. It can also help decrease depression, brain fog, and fatigue.

Instead of IV treatments, I may also inject ozone into trigger points, particularly in the muscles of the back and other injured areas.

A former pro football player recently visited me. He'd had surgery on a ruptured Achilles tendon that wasn't healing after six months of physical therapy. Still, his achilles would tighten every morning so much that he suffered with golfing, walking, and football. I injected PRP and ozone around his Achilles tendon. Two days later, he called me elated as he was able to play a round of golf and walked the entire course.

Ozone works quickly because you receive immediate oxygen to the area of injury. Muscle tissue, especially trigger points, lack blood flow and oxygen. As it loses that blood flow and oxygen, it becomes tight (a point of fibrosis and pain) until you break up that tissue and re-oxygenate it. Instead of dry-needling, injecting steroids (which can make the muscle weaker), or lidocaine (which only masks the pain without helping the injury), by receiving regenerative therapies like

PRP and ozone you may experience true healing of the tissue— instead of just a cover up.

I try to give ozone to most patients getting PRP and exosomes[8]. When I inject a muscle, joint, or orthopedic condition, the person usually feels better that day when they walk out of my office.

Scream Cream

Scream Cream contains a generic form of Viagra (a vasodilator for increased blood flow), DHEA (which acts to improve the tissue health), and testosterone. My compounding pharmacist creates tailor-made cream that includes a tasteless base to carry the ingredients into the tissue. Then, 10 to 30 minutes before sexual relations, you apply the cream to the clitoris and vagina. Patients use the cream when they want more desire and enhanced arousal.

It causes an ***"erection" of the clitoris*** due to the vasodilation within the tissue of the clitoris from the generic Viagra. The testosterone combined with DHEA and generic Viagra will often intensify a woman's orgasm, especially if she applies it to the clitoris and the G-spot. Almost every woman who gets a Scream Cream prescription will want a refill.

The Love Hormone

Oxytocin is a hormone peptide that is naturally produced by the Hypothalamus. It is called the "Love Drug" and I call it the "Pepe Le Pew" drug. If you have a hard time bonding with your partner and or if you experience issues with love, connection, or arousal with sexual intercourse, oxytocin can help tremendously. If you're not secreting enough oxytocin, you can struggle with feeling like your emotions are flat and oxytocin can help some people feel more connected to their lover and more aroused.

A big part of arousal and sexual intercourse is the connection with your lover. ***We get oxytocin naturally through breastfeeding, stimulation of nipples, or hugs lasting longer than eight seconds.*** Many of us are deficient in this love hormone because we are on our phones and computers, and most recently social distancing, instead of interacting face-to-face with other people.

Oxytocin, "the cuddle hormone", is excreted in large quantities at birth to help a mother bond with her baby. You'll see ads in men's magazines mentioning oxytocin cologne. You're supposed to put it on and women supposedly fall in love with you, but these contain minuscule amounts of oxytocin; but, that's the theory behind those products. With a proper administration of a prescription strength oxytocin, the effects can be amazing.

We administer oxytocin in three ways:

1. Injecting with a small "insulin" needle, daily, or as wanted for connection, love and sex.
2. As a nasal spray[3], which can be used every day to increase human connection, bonding, or intercourse (this delivery method works the fastest).
3. As a troche (under the tongue), 30 to 60 minutes prior to intercourse. With this method, you have to be careful to not swallow— if you do, the stomach will digest the hormone before it can be absorbed.

Recently, a young mother came to see me who even as a mom felt disconnected from her children and family; a recent struggle with depression, divorce, and a job change left her feeling emotionally flat and isolated. So, I put her on a *custom-designed, daily oxytocin regimen. After two weeks on oxytocin, she felt the "bonding"* return. Oxytocin also gave her energy. She pulled her life together, had energy, and felt great about herself— due to the newfound bonding and normal human interactions again.

Oxytocin will not cause human bonding to occur where such bonding is undeserved— it's not a magic potion that makes you fall in love with just anyone. But, the hormone does *allow you to respond with the appropriately earned emotions that should come when you experience affection from others.*

Defeat the Silent Torturer, Lichen Sclerosus

My primary focus for the past twelve years has been women's health in family medicine, functional medicine, aesthetics, and regenerative medicine. One of the more severe challenges that face women is lichen sclerosus, which can cause bleeding and pain in the areas of the vagina that instead should experience pleasure.

To treat both lichen sclerosus or the extreme vaginal dryness that happens after radiation or chemotherapy, I inject directly into the damaged tissue of the vagina or vulva. That accomplishes the regeneration of collagen and neovascularization and down-regulates the autoimmune response.

As an example, I had been treating a 46-year-old woman who suffered with autoimmune problems for six months before she finally admitted to me that she suffered from lichen sclerosus. She was embarrassed by the associated shame, fear, and other severely negative emotions that often plague the women who suffer with this disease.

My own patient was embarrassed to talk to me, her physician, about her vaginal dryness; such shame and fear about the conversation is common with women who suffer with sexual problems. Often, women have been berated or ignored when they brought up the issue with previous physicians; so they simply choose to suffer in silence.

Before finding me, because of severe sclerosus, this woman had suffered a tear to her vagina during a routine pelvic exam. Her physician did not listen to her; so, she greatly feared undergoing another pap smear or even to visit a gynecologist. This scenario happens way too often. She had been visiting me for other issues for 6 months before sharing this experience.

Her lichen sclerosus caused her to itch and bleed when she simply urinated. She would tear when she wiped after urinating. That's brutally dry. On blood testing, she had practically zero estrogen. A vaginal exam was almost impossible because she suffered such profound dryness and pain.

She had never been married nor had children due to her "PTSD" related to these issues from prior relationships. Can you imagine the pain of that?

She had not been diagnosed or followed by her dermatologist or gynecologist. Nobody was treating her, even though she had a severe rash that itches and caused severe pain. She'd seen one or two primary care doctors when she was younger. She was finally tested years later when much of the scarring disappeared. The biopsy came back: lichen sclerosus.

In primary care, as I was initially trained, there wasn't much I could do to help her other than give steroids that cause other unwanted side effects. But with new cellular therapies in functional medicine, I changed her life.

After we first spoke, she agreed to a pap smear. I also gave her an O-Shot® procedure and added specific PRP injections to the vulvar area where she had lesions and scarring all the way to the rectum. She also suffered with difficulty with bowel movements; so, I injected the entire perineum and around the rectum.

Eight weeks later, she experienced a life-changing improvement. She got into a relationship and visited an OBGYN to get her women's health needs addressed. Nine months later, she was still having love and sex. I haven't had to retreat her with any other lichen treatments.

With men, I can see similar results by focusing on cellular therapies that affect the function of the tissues. For example, I treated a man who had suffered through a prostatectomy as a treatment for his prostate cancer. He's in his 70's and is married to a healthy 47-year-old woman. He hadn't had an erection in four years. Doctors didn't cut any nerves, but they at least nicked one because he had no erection after his prostatectomy.

The first time I injected him with the P-Shot® combined with exosomes and he saw a 50% improvement. After six months, I added shockwave therapy to the P-Shot® and exosomes. I also gave him PT-141 for use prior to intercourse to help with blood flow and arousal.

He's now at 90% function for getting and maintaining an erection. He takes Cialis daily, plus PT-141 as needed for intercourse. He's very happy, has his sexual function back, and experiences full erections now with his deepening relationship with his wife.

Synergistic Results from Combined Cellular and Regenerative Therapies

Usually, women love the first O-Shot® procedure, but we often repeat it every 9 to 18 months to maintain or improve the effects. As mentioned, I often add ozone, exosomes, amnion, and/or Wharton's Jelly for outstanding results.

Other problems involving remodeling of tissue, like scarring of the face from acne or the body from surgery can be treated. For example, amnion mixed with exosomes or PRP works great to reduce scars. Yesterday, I treated a young female patient with a large sternotomy scar from a previous surgery. First, I pretreated the area with radiofrequency micro-needling. Then I injected and applied topical PRP and amnion in the area. I also sent her home with a formulated mix of topical exosomes, growth factors, hyaluronic acid, vitamins and amino acids to improve healing and results. *These combination therapies give a synergistic effect that can often be amazing.*

When I treat scars with microneedling only versus adding cellular therapy to the microneedling, there's absolutely no comparison. One woman whom I recently treated with microneedling followed by PRP and exosomes for acne and an abscess, actually texted me a few days later and said, "I'm not kidding you, my scars are already better."

I offer these treatments for *acne scars, surgical scars, lichen sclerosus or almost any type of scar.*

I have also had great results treating patients with **Peyronie's disease (a form of scarring of the penis that causes pain and a crooked erection)**. When treating Peyronie's disease, I also often add exosomes, ozone, and shockwave.

Other synergistic effects can be seen when you add CBD to natural lubricants like coconut oil. **CBD can cause clitoral enlargement naturally and increase orgasm. Adding CBD enhances arousal, sensation, and orgasm.**

Unfortunately, many men and women who find their way to me have suffered much shame and discouragement about their disease. I relate due to the battles with my own health that I have fought and won and because of the thousands of people I have helped. The good news that many cellular and regenerative therapies are now available that can change lives: the O-Shot®, the P-Shot®, exosomes, amnion, oxytocin, ozone, PT-141, and CBD oil. You do not have to remain stuck where you are; often, a combination of regenerative treatments can change your life and the life of those who love you.

Steps to Your Sexual Wellness

1. Vaginal dryness is common but treatable. *Do not settle for continued pain.* Talk with your doctor to get the right treatment.

2. *Speak with your physician about sexual issues,* so they can help you or refer you to an expert who can. Insist on persistent pursuit of your healing with your personal physician as your guide and consider the various cellular therapies as an option.

3. Treatments are available to increase your quality of life. You can try many different options. Find the right one for you.

4. A good skincare regimen can help hydrate your vaginal tissues, don't settle for simply thinking about your face!

More About Dr. Cristyn Watkins

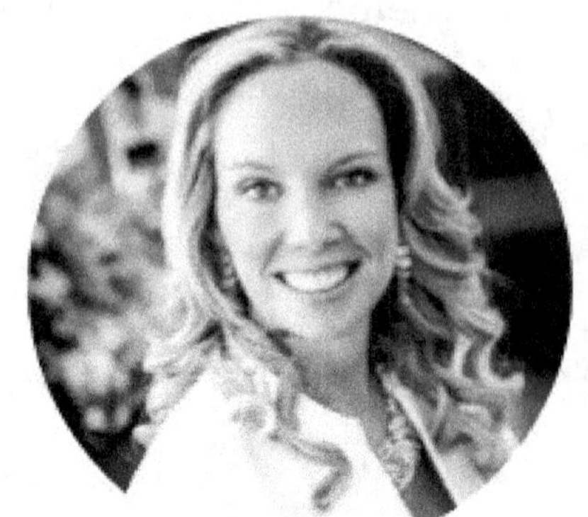

Dr. Cristyn Watkins has been the visionary, owner, and medical director of aNu Aesthetics and Optimal Wellness since 2011, with two locations in Kansas City, Missouri.

She is double board certified in Family Medicine and Functional/Metabolic/Nutrition Medicine. She is a National Trainer for Allergan Aesthetics and CoolSculpting. She is trained in Medical Aesthetics, Laser and Body Contouring, Bio-Identical Hormones, Medical Weight Loss, Regenerative Medicine, and Functional Medicine.

Her recent passion in Regenerative Medicine has allowed her to focus a lot of her research and practice on advanced therapies such as Exosomes, Ozone, PRP, Peptides and IV Nutritional Therapy. She is a National Regenerative Medicine Trainer for Nurse Practitioners with RegenEd and is the owner of Regenerative Treatment Centers of Leawood, Kansas.

She has a desire to empower patients to take care of themselves on the inside and the outside with aesthetics, wellness and healthy aging and hopes all of her patients can achieve this lifestyle. She has treated chronic disease, pain, inflammation, autoimmune and immune disorders, weight problems, thyroid conditions, menstrual and hormone issues for over a decade. She has continued her extensive education and training to develop new treatments to overcome these conditions and has been very successful at helping patients achieve a healthier, happier, and younger self!

- Website: aNuAesthetics.com
- Location: Kansas City, Missouri, USA
- Phone: 816-359-3310

References

1. Ann N Y Acad Sci. 2003 Jun;994:96-102. PT-141: a melanocortin agonist for the treatment of sexual dysfunction. Molinoff PB1, Shadiack AM, Earle D, Diamond LE, Quon CY.

2. J Sex Med. 2006 Jul;3(4):628-638. doi: 10.1111/j.1743-6109.2006.00268.x. An effect on the subjective sexual response in premenopausal women with sexual arousal disorder by bremelanotide (PT-141), a melanocortin receptor agonist. Diamond LE1,

Earle DC2, Heiman JR3, Rosen RC4, Perelman MA5, Harning R1.

3. Int J Impot Res. 2004 Feb;16(1):51-9. Double-blind, placebo-controlled evaluation of the safety, pharmacokinetic properties and pharmacodynamic effects of intranasal PT-141, a melanocortin receptor agonist, in healthy males and patients with mild-to-moderate erectile dysfunction. Diamond LE1, Earle DC, Rosen RC, Willett MS, Molinoff PB.

4. Stem Cell Res Ther. 2018 Sep 26;9(1):246. doi: 10.1186/s13287-018-1003-1. MSC-derived exosomes ameliorate erectile dysfunction by alleviation of corpus cavernosum smooth muscle apoptosis in a rat model of cavernous nerve injury. Ouyang X1, Han X2, Chen Z1, Fang J1, Huang X2, Wei H3.

5. Andrology. 2018 Nov;6(6):927-935. doi: 10.1111/andr.12519. Epub 2018 Jul 16. Exosomes derived from mesenchymal stem cells exert therapeutic effect in a rat model of cavernous nerves injury. Li M1, Lei H2, Xu Y3, Li H1, Yang B1, Yu C4, Yuan Y1, Fang D1, Xin Z1, Guan R1.

6. J Cell Mol Med. 2019 Nov;23(11):7462-7473. doi: 10.1111/jcmm.14615. Epub 2019 Sep 11. Mesenchymal stem cell-derived exosomes ameliorate erection by reducing oxidative stress damage of corpus cavernosum in a rat model of artery injury. Liu Y1, Zhao S1,2, Luo L1, Wang J1, Zhu Z1, Xiang Q1, Deng Y1, Zhao Z1.

7. IV ozone:
   - https://www.ncbi.nlm.nih.gov/pmc/articles/PMC6178636/
   - https://www.ncbi.nlm.nih.gov/pmc/articles/PMC5674660/

8. Ozone for muscle pain/back pain/orthopedic:
   - https://www.ncbi.nlm.nih.gov/pmc/articles/PMC6178642/
   - https://www.ncbi.nlm.nih.gov/pubmed/29633741
   - https://www.ncbi.nlm.nih.gov/pmc/articles/PMC4523667/

Chapter 4:
Build Confidence
Using Male Augmentation
by Dr. Bill Song

Is male augmentation even a thing? Consider for a moment how the concept of penile enhancement compares to breast augmentation. Twenty years ago, breast implants were taboo, not something any "normal" woman might consider. Now, breast enlargement with implants are mainstream.

Imagine if male augmentation followed this same trend. I would imagine the beach and pool scene might get a little different (a lot more Speedos).

Like it or not, I believe there is a new trend starting. ***Once more men discover that there is a safe and effective way to make it happen, penile enlargement procedures may become one of the fastest growing trends in cosmetic surgery.*** Men who have had the procedure absolutely love it and most come back for second, third or more sessions. I have had to refuse further enhancements for some of my patients because I am afraid it will start looking abnormal. Once they discover this "fountain of huge", men absolutely love the feeling it gives them. One of my patients has actually described it as "life-changing!"

My first male augmentation patient came in for a consultation with his wife in 2012. After listening to both the man and his wife, I was puzzled. What were his reasons? This man claimed he was loyal to his wife, and his wife was not complaining. In fact, what she said to me was, "I don't know why he wants this. I am perfectly happy with his penis. He is not small."

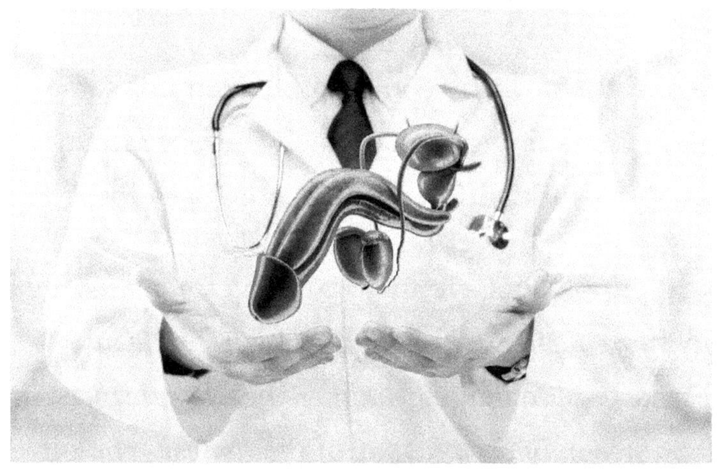

When I asked the patient himself, he told me, "I'm not doing this for anyone else. This procedure is for me."

Then I remembered hearing many women tell me the same thing about having breast implants, "This procedure is for me, not to impress anyone else." So, in the same way, the first man to receive penile augmentation from me wasn't trying to impress a woman or to one up his buddies; he simply felt that male augmentation would increase his confidence, and it did! He was so happy with the procedure that he started recommending it to his friends. Soon my cosmetic medicine practice, which previously catered almost exclusively to women, was getting a steady stream of men coming in for this novel procedure. When I first decided to go into medicine, I never would have imagined that this is what I would be doing, but this is the story of how I became "Dr. Hung."

A penis is not outwardly visible like breasts on a woman, so why are men so self conscious about their size? Why is it so important for some men to have a big penis? There are the obvious reasons like, to impress their sexual partner or impress their peers in the locker room, or even for the unlikely chance that someone might call them out when they brag about it.

These are all valid reasons men want to have an enhancement procedure, but I think it runs much deeper than that. Think about how our culture insinuates penis size with so many other things. For example, if a man drives a fancy car or is overly arrogant, he "must have a small penis and is compensating for it." Even during a recent U.S. presidential primary, back-handed insults were exchanged with one candidate claiming small hands meant small "something else," and the other candidate actually feeling the need to publicly defend himself against the allegation. Imagine a man watching a movie with his spouse or partner and the requisite, gratuitous nudity scene pops on the screen. These days, it's not just breasts. Full frontal displays of exceptionally well hung male actors are becoming commonplace in movies and on cable television.

Caught off guard, the woman makes an almost imperceptible gasp. That could knock down a man's self confidence for the evening or maybe even for the rest of his life!

This is the reality of the society we live in. Just like women do with their breast size, men have to muster up enough self-confidence to be happy with themselves regardless of what society tells them...

Oh wait, what year is it? Yes, that's right, let's get real. Nobody today is going to settle for their natural endowment when a simple in-office treatment can offer them bigger and more! That is the reality we live in. Having a bigger penis is not actually going to make you more successful or more alpha, but if you have the ways and means, you now have the option to choose between a new sports car or a bigger penis.

If people are going to do it anyway, I can offer a way to do it safely without risking complications and disfigurement. As a doctor, I am always leaning towards the more conservative approach, but as an artist, I welcome the challenge of being creative. *I see the human body as a canvas where I can create magnificent, yet natural looking faces, breasts, buttocks, abs and yes, even penises.*

The "Micro Penis" Stigma

I constantly get calls from guys who think they have a "Micro Penis." Just the fact that this terminology even exists is enough to terrify some men who actually would be considered quite normal in size. Occasionally, I do get some men who actually have what is clinically considered a micro penis.

For an adult male to be considered as having a micro penis, the stretched length needs to be less than 3.67 inches. The average, by the way, is 5.21 inches, NOT 8 inches as I was led to believe by the braggers in high school. The stretched length is determined by stretching the penis as far as it will go, measuring from base to the tip. This length is about the same length as when the penis is erect.

Most men are surprised to learn that the average penile length is much smaller than they thought. There are several reasons why this is. Men like to brag and exaggerate. One common phrase heard around the locker room is "I'm a grower, not a shower." This is making reference to the fact that flaccid size does not necessarily correlate to erect size and insinuating that their erect size is much bigger. The typical claims are 8, 9, and even 10 inches when erect.

Then there are the actual "showers" (as in show-er – one who shows, as opposed to "taking a shower"). We had a guy on our college track team whose nickname was "Tripod." He was definitely a "shower." And he certainly liked to show it. He was always "hanging" out in the locker room naked, making sure everyone saw how well endowed he was. These types of encounters and others, like witnessing scenes from the stolen Tommy Lee and Pamela Anderson videos can be traumatizing to a young man trying to access his own manhood. I'm only half joking here.

There are men who do actually suffer from a penis that is too small to the point that it interferes with sexual function. One such patient of mine had a normal length but the girth was the issue. When I first spoke to him on the phone, he described his penis as a lollipop, a normal sized head but with a very thin shaft. In this case, his wife was not happy with his size since ***it was difficult for her to feel him inside of her.*** He was the perfect person to treat with fillers combined with a P-Shot® procedure. We were able to more than double his girth, and made it not only look normal, but function normally as well.

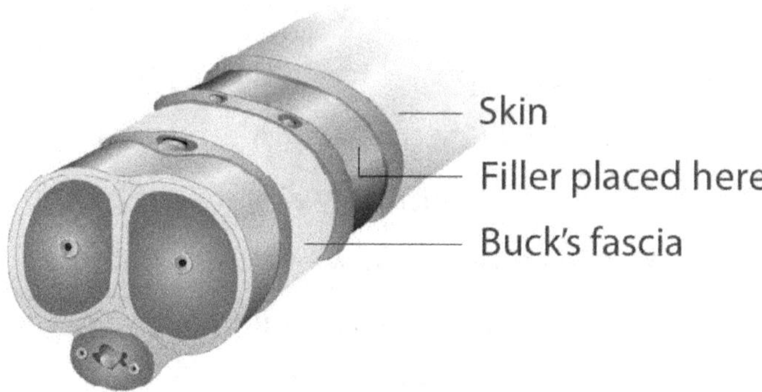

After two rounds, his **marriage** improved. He said that he felt his wife respected him more. If you are self-conscious about your penis size then any statement a partner makes is easy to second-guess. Without a shred of evidence, many men with smaller penises suspect their partners of cheating on them and often make accusations that could eventually become a self-fulfilling prophecy. *Wives tell me their husbands are easier to live with after the treatment because they are not as sensitive about the issue.*

Avoiding the "Gimmicks"

Ever since I can remember, penis growth pills were a popular gimmick. Before the internet, the classified ads section of Rolling Stone magazine was where you could typically find advertisements for pills and creams to enhance your manhood. Now, these advertisements are so common on the internet that even my wife complains about all the spam emails she gets promising to increase HER penis size. Men are very skeptical because they have been bombarded with gimmicks and scams. Many have probably been "had," sometimes more than once, and are now understandably jaded. These days, the promise of penis size growth equals "scam" for many people. It is a challenge for me to even let people know that there are valid medical treatments that actually work. The scammers are still out there, but now we have real treatments that actually work.

The trick is to find legitimate doctors who know what they are doing. Be careful! There are some serious complications that can easily be avoided by well trained doctors, but cheap, fly by night operations are common and they can really mess up your stuff. There are reputable clinics overseas and some of them are actually more advanced than what is typically available in the States, but if you reside in the US and have it done in a foreign country, you may not have any recourse if there is a complication.

Some US doctors set up clinics over the border to avoid FDA oversight. Wherever you decide to have the procedure done, you must do your due diligence. These procedures are not cheap. Large amounts of fillers are often needed to achieve the desired result, so it is understandable that some men will choose the clinic based on the lowest prices they are quoted.

The statement, "If it sounds too good to be true, it probably is..." is very true in the arena of penile enhancement. As you make your decisions about where and by whom you want to have the procedure done, *you should also seriously consider the option of not doing it at all.*

Penis Possibilities

Do this for the right reasons. Understand your options— including the option of doing nothing. Most men who undergo penile augmentation are not "small" before the procedure. It is not about "becoming" normal. ***Research shows that most women are happy with their partner's penis size.***

We can change girth, and flaccid penile length, but there are not many great options to increase erect length. With girth enhancement, the extra weight of the penis will cause it to hang lower while flaccid. There will be extra girth when erect but the maximum length will remain the same. The glans (head) can be enlarged with temporary fillers. Permanent fillers are not recommended in the head. There are a variety of ways we can increase the girth of your penis. The products named below are FDA cleared for use in the face. Injections into the penis are considered "off label."

Here are some of your choices:

- Doing ***nothing***. You are fine how you are.
- ***Priapus Shot®*** procedure; also known as the P-Shot® procedure— a regenerative treatment

113

using platelet-rich plasma (PRP) to give a modest increase in natural growth.

- *Testosterone* can increase penis size in some men but can cause testicular atrophy.

- *Surgical* options. An implant or cylinder can be placed to treat severe erectile dysfunction. There are many complications but still most men are happy with the outcome and the size increase that comes with the procedure.

- *Penuma*® is a sleeve that can be placed under the skin of the penis. This involves surgery and is a permanent implant.

- *Dermal hyaluronic acid (HA) fillers* (like Juvederm®, Restylane® and Versa®) combined with a Priapus Shot® procedure. This doesn't require an operating room. Fillers are simple. No ligaments are cut, and no surgery is needed. However, be careful. There can still be complications. If done correctly, it's a simple procedure that takes ten minutes and can last a year, and it is reversible if you don't love it.

- *Collagen stimulating fillers.* Products like Radiesse®, Sculptra® and Bellafill® are in a class of collagen stimulators. These can give you longer lasting volume, with PMMA based products like Bellafill® giving potentially permanent results. I will talk more about PMMA below.

- A *vacuum pump* increases size, especially after a P-Shot®. *Stretching devices* can be awkward to use, and you must be careful not to be overzealous, but they can also help.

PMMA: An Injectable Implant

PMMA Poly(methyl methacrylate) PMMA is a synthetic material that has been used as medical and dental implants since the 1940's. Because of its remarkable biocompatibility, PMMA is one of the most common materials used in making medical implants such as pacemakers, joint replacements and even lens replacement for the eye. A novel use of PMMA in cosmetic medicine is the micro implants. These are tiny microscopic beads that are small enough to be injected with a needle or cannula. When injected into the skin, these beads act as a scaffold for collagen to form around. The process is similar to a coral reef forming around rocks or a sunken ship.

Some of my patients have traveled to Mexico for a massive dose (30ccs or more) of generic PMMA and have severe deformities as a result. Many doctors fear these complications and so won't use PMMA at all. But, when I use PMMA, I use the Bellafill® brand and I do multiple treatments with small amounts of PMMA to decrease the risk of nodules. I typically inject no more than 5ccs at a time. I also combine the PMMA with PRP (Platelet-Rich Plasma derived from your own blood). As with the Vampire Facelift® procedure, the PRP is activated by the presence of the filler and amplifies production of your own collagen. With both the face and the penis, less filler is needed to achieve the same results when we combine the filler with PRP. We routinely see a very robust regeneration of collagen with less risk of nodules. We finish the procedure with an acoustic wave treatment for further stimulation of collagen and to smooth everything into a beautiful natural shape. We greatly reduced the incidence of nodules by using this combination of PRP, plus PMMA, combined with shock wave therapy and always performing the work in stages, rather than all at once.

For patients who are reluctant to have permanent implants, there is also the option of using Sculptra® or PLLA (Poly-L-Lactic Acid). PLLA is the same material used in dissolvable sutures. It has the same collagen stimulating effect as PMMA but the actual particles dissolve away leaving the collagen shell which can last about two years. This is a nice "in-between" option compared to the permanent PMMA and the HA fillers that last about a year. I like to add PRP to any of the materials that I use because the growth factors from the PRP will amplify the effects.

When injecting Platelet-Rich Plasma or biologicals like exosomes and stem cells, I'll inject directly into the corpus cavernosum to achieve better circulation and improved erection with a possible decrease in venous leak. Fillers or fat should never be injected into the corpus. ***In case any doctors are reading this, the information presented here is to educate the public and is not meant as a how-to guide.*** Please get the proper training before attempting the treatment on your patients. I must reiterate, ***I never inject fillers or fat directly into the corpus cavernosum.***

Fat Transfers & Nano Fat—
A Part of Your Plan?

We can also perform fat transfers to the penis. The problem with fat is that your penis is the one area in your body where there is naturally no fat. It is hard to get fat to stay there. When we transfer fat into the penile shaft, it rarely stays and is often quickly absorbed away. When it does stay, it feels very pillowy. Some men describe it as having a down jacket on their penis.

Instead of trying to transfer intact fat cells, I now use *nano fat*, which has been processed to release growth factors and stem cells from the harvested fat. This helps with natural collagen formation and could influence natural growth in the area.

We get the best results with combination treatments: regenerative treatments, like P-Shot®, combined with dermal fillers and PRP along the shaft. We optimize hormones and sometimes add peptide therapies like PT141. We approach this not as a singular problem, but with the goal of an overall healthy sex life. People live longer lives now, having sex in later years, and are still conscious about the appearance of the face, body, and genitals. My goal is to enhance the sex lives of couples, no matter their age. It is not about vanity, it's about self-confidence and how they interact with each other. Many times, men discover my treatments because their wives come in for an O-Shot® or ThermiVa® treatment. The women are happy with their treatments and want their partners to be happy too. Not necessarily looking for their partner to be bigger. They want that partner to be happy with themselves and sometimes to improve genital matching.

Complications and Safety

Your safety is our primary concern. Yes, I know, everyone says that, but when we perform this type of "unconventional" treatment, any complication can become an extremely embarrassing situation for the patient and can be disastrous for the doctor's reputation. We are very cautious and conservative with our treatments. I prefer to do multiple sessions than one large session. It is much safer that way. ***Recently, a billionaire from France died*** from complications while having a penile augmentation procedure. Incidentally, his death was due to complications from the anesthesia, they had not even started the procedure on the penis, yet he will always be remembered as the guy who died while having a penis enlargement procedure. I can imagine how embarrassing this must be for his family. People can forget that there is a significant risk with general anesthesia.

We do not need to put anybody under general anesthesia for penile augmentation. Just topical and local anesthesia are all we need. Injecting into the wrong place can result in fillers or fat traveling through the blood vessels to the lungs which can result in a pulmonary embolism. This can be fatal and must be avoided at all costs. Fortunately, with a simple knowledge of the anatomy, this type of tragic complication can easily be avoided.

Infections are not common, but are always a risk especially when working in this area which tends to have lots of bacteria. We thoroughly clean the area with a surgical scrub and use sterile technique to avoid infection. Antibiotics are also given as a precautionary measure.

Nodules are not life threatening, but can be disfiguring. Nodule formation is the most common complication when augmenting the penis with any kind of filler. It can be particularly problematic when using a permanent product like PMMA. By performing the procedure in stages, using smaller amounts combined with PRP and using acoustic wave treatments to smooth and set the product, we have been able to achieve very nice results without nodule formation. We do have ways to shrink down nodules, but we much prefer to avoid them in the first place.

WARNING: PMMA administered in Mexico is usually not the FDA-cleared Bellafill®. The only PMMA injectable that I use for my procedures is Bellafill® because of the uniform size and smooth spherical shape of the particles. The size of the PMMA particles is important. If they're too small, the PMMA can be engulfed by the white blood cells and cause formation of a true granuloma which can be very difficult to treat. If the particles are too big, they can clump together and be palpable under the skin.

Too many times, cheap PMMA is injected in massive doses at a single visit, making it more likely that the man will suffer with unsightly nodules. If done improperly, intracavernous injections of fat or PMMA could lead to pulmonary emboli and death. This should be done by someone who knows what they are doing using high quality PMMA. The PRP preparation also needs to be performed using sterile technique and GTP standards, preferably with a quality FDA cleared kit.

Other risks include the loss of sensation. The presence of the filler does not usually cause loss of sensation unless massive amounts are injected. Typically, the loss of sensation that some men report is due to over aggressively using a vacuum pump on the penis. We routinely recommend a vacuum device after the procedures, but if men report their erections worsened after pumping, then often they pumped far beyond the recommended minus 5-10 mm of mercury that we recommend. The pump pressures should be carefully and individually prescribed by an experienced physician.

On the internet, I've seen people hanging weights from their penises. I would not recommend that. It does not seem safe. But, a carefully applied traction device made for the penis can sometimes be helpful.

It's difficult to gauge how aggressive you should be while stretching and pumping your penis. Be careful.

123

It's difficult to gauge how aggressive you should be while stretching and pumping your penis. Be careful.

A Smooth Take Off Into Better Sex

As with any medical treatment, your visit to my clinic would begin with questions about your medical history to ensure you were a good candidate. Active heart issues or uncontrolled medical conditions such as diabetes could disqualify you from treatment. We want you to be at your optimal health when we perform this procedure. We also want to make sure that you are capable and willing to follow our after care instructions. Our aftercare instructions are simple: Finish your antibiotics, keep the areas clean and massage as instructed. Use the pump as instructed. Abstain from sex until the entry sites are healed (usually 2-3 days).

This is significantly less risky than procedures where general anesthesia is involved. Nevertheless, we take every precaution to avoid having you end up in the emergency room with a complication. Imagine having to explain to nurses at the hospital about the procedure that you just had done.

Our society has not yet evolved to accept a penile enhancement complication in the same way as a breast implant issue. I would hope that hospitals and medical professionals abide by HIPAA patient privacy but the gossip mill can be brutal. We want zero complications with this because even a minor complication could lead to people finding out about the man having the procedure and can be quite humiliating.

Our staff are familiar with patients coming in for erectile dysfunction and penile enhancement procedures. Patients email me directly. Many come from referrals and they all have my email address for direct communication. I have a web page that answers frequent questions, shows before-and-afters, and lists prices. When men visit for these procedures, they already know exactly what's involved and what they want.

Many times, if my staff senses hesitation over the phone, they'll say, "I'll have Dr. Song call you back." Then, I speak to that possible future patient directly. They do not need to have a conversation with anyone else. I have mostly female staff. They are very professional and familiar with what we do, but they understand that men may not be comfortable talking about this sensitive subject with them. On the flip side, some men feel more comfortable having a female doctor work on them in this area. Others would rather go somewhere out of state where there is no chance of running into a staff member who may know them. Not a problem, I have trained many doctors around the country and can refer you to very competent and professional colleagues.

Sometimes, we face unrealistic expectations. It is not uncommon for me to tell a patient that he has had enough. I will not make a man look like a monster no matter how much he begs me to do it. If you have had other procedures and already have an implant, this may disqualify you from having the treatment due to the risk of infecting that implant.

The Procedure: Exactly What Happens With Your Penis

First, we ask that you shave your genitals the night before, so we don't have to work around the hair. After electronic and HIPAA compliant paperwork is completed, we clean you very well with Hibiclens®, a surgical scrub. We apply a strong topical numbing agent, and while that takes effect, we draw blood to get Platelet-Rich Plasma. As the PRP is spinning and being prepared, we make sure that all of your questions are answered and we go over post-procedure instructions. We make sure you are perfectly numbed.

Men are understandably afraid that doing "work" in this area will hurt. But, with the proper topical numbing cream, the procedure is not as painful as you may think. The skin gets nice and numb. We can also perform a nerve block with an injection if you want it to be completely numb.

First, I administer the Priapus Shot® to enhance the circulation and natural growth potential of the penis. Then I use a blunt tipped cannula to inject filler into the shaft. This is where the artistry comes in. I inject it evenly so it is smooth, not lumpy or lopsided. After the filler is injected, I add PRP and then smooth it out with an acoustic wave device. The shock waves make a big difference in making it come out smoothly. The challenge is to ensure that all of the material is placed in an aesthetically proportional manner to create an enlarged but normal appearing shape.

I am careful where I inject the materials, being mindful of blood vessels. I stay superficial to the Buck's fascia. I stay away from the corpus cavernosum. The trick is not to use a cannula that is too thin. Many doctors and injectors mistakenly think the smaller cannulas are safer. Smaller cannulas are more like needles because they are small and sharp. Larger, wider cannulas are safer. We use a cannula, which is not likely to pierce a blood vessel.

I've done enough of these procedures that I can do it very quickly in 10 minutes. It might take a new doctor an hour or more to ensure they get it right. After the injection, we use an acoustic sound wave device to smooth out the fillers. We do not need to apply a cast or tight bandages because the product is "set" by the acoustic wave treatment and unlikely to migrate.

Years ago, I began administering *GainsWave®* *(acoustic shock waves)* to improve the firmness of erection. Now, I also use the acoustic waves to smooth out the material injected for augmentation. The shock wave device works like a motorized tamper that contractors use to smooth out the gravel before laying asphalt on your driveway. The goal is a nice, smooth finish.

For many procedures, like a surgical implant, you must wait a month before having sex. Our procedures only require 2 days of waiting. The reason to wait: we want the small needle holes to close. We don't want bacteria getting in there when you have sex.

The patient is instructed to use a vacuum penis pump after the treatment. Before the procedure, we ensure we are using the proper size cylinder for the penis pump. We don't want it so small that it doesn't fit you, but we want it small enough that the sides of the penis are fully in contact when inflated against the cylinder. That helps to form the final result. We fit you to a cylinder size that might feel a little tight. This is so we can mold the material along the sides of the cylinder. We can always move you to a larger diameter tube later, if needed.

Frequently Asked Questions

Q: Is it painful?

A: We use local anesthesia. The area is completely numb and you are fully awake. Patients sometimes get nervous with a procedure on the penis. We can use Pro-Nox or nitrous oxide to help you relax. I rarely use sedatives as they are unnecessary when I do the procedure.

Q: Which filler product do you recommend?

A: Hyaluronic acid fillers are the safest because they are reversible if you do not like the way it looks, but they are temporary. The results may last 6 months to a year. PMMA is more long lasting. The microspheres are permanent but the FDA allows the company to claim 5 years for Bellafill® since that is how long the patients were followed in the studies. Other PMMA products are not cleared for use in the United States. Fat transfer to the penis can give you the most volume but the fat does not tend to stay very well in this area. PLLA or Sculptra® is an "in between" option. Results can last two years after a series of 2-3 treatments. I like to combine any of these procedures with a P-Shot®, which helps with natural growth.

Q: How much does it cost?

A: In order to get a noticeable improvement, the initial treatment will require injecting enough material to give you a nice base. This will cost around $6000. Subsequent treatments will vary depending on how much additional product is injected and the cost will be between $1800 to $6000. The best thing to do would be to schedule a personal consultation so we can give you an accurate estimate. Warning: Penis enlargement can be addicting. If you are looking for massive volume, it could easily cost you tens of thousands of dollars.

Q: Do you need to be circumcised to have the procedure?

A: This procedure can be performed on circumcised and uncircumcised men. In uncircumcised men, the trick is not to put too much at the distal end of the foreskin, otherwise, the head will not protrude out, almost like phimosis.

Q: Can you enlarge the head?

A: The head of the penis is more difficult to enlarge. We can inject hyaluronic acid fillers in the glands but I do not inject PMMA or fat because you can lose sensation and scar tissue can form. Instead, I like to add an extra amount of PRP or biologicals like exosomes or stem cell products. Because we are limited in the type of products we can use, any enlargement to the head is usually temporary.

Q: Do I need to wrap the penis after the procedure?

A: Certain providers, especially when using PMMA, wrap the penis in a "cast" for days to help form the shape, and to keep the product from settling distally. For that reason, Bellafill® is suspended in collagen as opposed to water, and therefore, it is less likely to settle and move. To prevent it from settling distally, we use smaller amounts and use an acoustic wave to set it. I do not wrap it.

Super Results

Size is not everything. Performance and mental attitude play a vital role in virility. In addition to the enhancement, a P-Shot®, exosomes, or a similar biological fertilizer, combined with some bioidentical testosterone replacement (if needed) may just give you a super-penis that you can be very proud of.

About Dr. Hung William Song

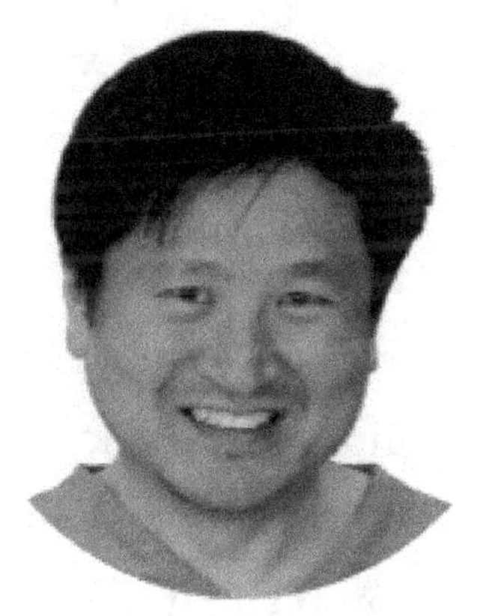

Dr. Song is a leading provider of laser and energy-based cosmetic treatments. He is a faculty trainer for the American Cosmetic and Cellular Medicine Association and the Advanced Aesthetics Education Group. He is a founding member of the American Academy of Stem Cell Physicians. He speaks around the country and teaches other doctors from around the world about PRP, stem cell treatments and advanced laser techniques.

- Website: P-ShotNJ.com
- Location: Oakland, New Jersey, USA
- Phone: 201-368-3800

Chapter 5:
Erectile Dysfunction
& Peyronie's Disease
by Dr. Dan Botha

Have you ever felt uncomfortable discussing "something" sensitive with your doctor, even when in private? 80% of men who suffer with ED never discuss their problem with a physician. *52% of men suffer from erectile dysfunction (ED)*; of these men, 57% are between the ages of 40 and 60.

Men often avoid discussing ED not only because of embarrassment but also because they think there may not be a solution. Some avoid the discussion because they think that since ED is not a life-threatening problem, it does not warrant attention by their physician. But, the World Health Organization states that health entails complete physical, mental, and social well-being, not merely the absence of disease and infirmity. And to feel confident and fully healthy, men need to function sexually.

When your body suffers suboptimal performance, you should always find the root cause— not just treat the symptoms. The main causes of ED include neurological, vascular, psychological, and hormonal. Neurological causes include multiple sclerosis, prostatectomy, and degenerative diseases such as spinal cord or nerve injuries or diabetes. Nerve damage can also come from surprising sources such as biking long distances and trauma. Vascular causes include poor blood flow associated with hypertension, vascular disease, endothelial damage, diabetes, and hypercholesterolemia. Psychological problems that cause ED include stress, depression, performance anxiety, unhealthy diet with associated lethargy, financial worry, and relationship/marriage discord.

Erectile dysfunction treatments cost men five billion dollars a year in the US alone; and ED can cause men to suffer much more than sexual problems— depression, loss of creativity and motivation (which leads to financial distress), broken relationships, and divorce with separation from young children all plague the man with ED.

Due to increasingly more stressful lifestyles— the ravages of modern existence (with unhealthy diet and sedentary habits), ED will only become more widespread. Hopefully, men will grow increasingly bolder about seeking root-cause solutions to their ED problem.

As the ***medical director of a busy erectile dysfunction clinic in Calgary, Alberta, Canada***, I have helped many men improve their sex, including most every underlying cause and its treatment.

A Menu of Treatments for ED

Most men find their best sexual function with a ***synergistic, tailor-made, combination*** of one or more of the following therapies.

Pharmaceutical

Until recently, the most commonly used treatments for ED were the **pharmaceutical agents**: *yohimbine, papaverine, phentolamine, atropine, and intracavernous injections like Bimix and Trimix*. Many men find help with the *PDE5 inhibitors like Viagra, Cialis, and Levitra*. All of these pharmaceutical treatments can cause side effects that for most men are tolerable but for some men can just be too uncomfortable (headache) or too dangerous (stroke or heart attack). Also, none of these treatments actually correct the underlying cause of the ED; they only compensate by helping residual tissue work harder. All of these agents can be used safely when prescribed strategically by someone who knows what they are doing; but there are multiple very good reasons why they are by prescription only.

Tissue Regenerative Agents

The next and *more modern class* of treatments for ED can actually help to *correct the underlying pathology*. A salamander can regrow a limb; imagine applying that same science to the penis! If we use this idea and we know that blood flow is one of the main reasons for erectile function, we can design regenerative therapies in the future.

For example, **with platelet-rich plasma (PRP)** administered by the specific method called the **P-Shot® (Priapus Shot®)**, we know that growth factors and cytokines from platelets can remodel scar tissue, improve blood flow, and rejuvenate nerve tissue. One study showed that the P-Shot® can in some men have a positive outcome with a venous leak. This procedure, which has become very popular, involves a simple blood draw from the man's arm, followed by using a specific centrifuge to isolate the PRP. We activate the PRP with Calcium Chloride and reinject it back into the penis. We block the penis with local anesthetics so there is no pain when the activated PRP is reinjected. The process takes 30-45 minutes to do.

We usually combine the P-Shot® with a **Nitric Oxide Stimulant like AFFIRM®** and a **vacuum pump protocol.** Penis pumps have been shown to increase the oxygen and blood flow level within the penis and to help correct scar tissue from Peyronie's disease and even to contribute to an increase in size in some men. As a well known urologist, Dr. Lee, in our town, said, "What you do not use you lose."

Penis vacuum pumps can enhance the effectiveness of both the P-Shot® and of the pharmaceutical agents.

Low-intensity extracorporeal shockwave therapy is another regenerative cellular therapy that has been used for the treatment of tendon injuries but now specific protocols have been designed for the penis. These protocols, like the GAINSWave protocols, can also improve blood flow and help remodel scar tissue to improve erection quality. The GAINSWave protocols work much better when combined with the P-Shot® protocol.

Future newer therapies to improve tissue health include **exosomes** from placenta and amnion fluid.

Exosomes are cell derivative vesicles that are a million times smaller than the diameter of a hair. Exosomes contain messenger RNA which is present in all biological fluids and carries growth factors like VNP7, DGF, and FGF-7 for cell growth and tissue repair as well as anti-inflammatory agents like DNP1 and DNP2. Exosomes most commonly come from amniotic products and we use concentrations of 50 billion exosomes per milliliter.

Exosomes do not contain the nuclear material seen with stem cells— making exosomes less worrisome. The source of exosomes being young amniotic tissue, it can provide better results when combined with PRP, since the PRP is as old as the donor who is being treated (it's his PRP from his blood, but the amnion comes from very young tissue).

Peptides are naturally occurring substances that form when two or more single amino acids join together via peptide bonds to form a short chain. Synthetic melanotropic peptides initiate erections in men with psychogenic erectile dysfunction. Similar effects on libido are seen in women. **Bremelanotide PT141** is a derivative of melanotan 2. It is a potent initiator of erections with minimal side effects. It has strong binding to MC receptors 1.3 and 4. Using 1 mg sc abdominal has notable effects 90 to 120 minutes after injections. Do not use with PD-5 inhibitors like Cialis.

Technologies to Improve Individual Treatment Strategies

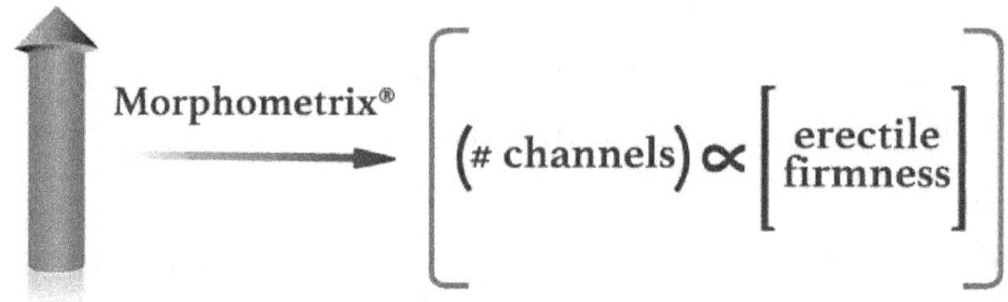

An increased number of open channels with Morphometrix scanning correlates with increased firmness.

The most simple and traditional way to measure ED treatment effectiveness is the SHIM score; you answer five questions, each question on a scale from one to five. So, your maximum score is 25 and the lowest score is 5.

The rating works as follows:

- 1-7 equals severe ED
- 8-11 means moderate ED
- 12-16 is mild-to-moderate ED
- 17-21 is mild ED

This simple scoring system, from 5 to 25, continues to serve doctors and patients as a way to measure treatment effectiveness. Doppler flow and ultrasound imaging provide a more exact way to both look at the penis and to measure effectiveness of treatment.

Working with a physicist, we formed a company, Morphometrix, to develop an even better method to both measure results and to design more tailor-made treatments for ED. We have been doing in-house ultrasounds using a handheld device, called Butterfly IQ. We scan both Corpus Covernosus and upload the MP4 image to our In-Cloud software, Morphometrix, where we look at the liquid interfaces in tissue.

This technology was originally created to look at damaged and torn tendons in racing horses since a horse cannot fit into an MRI machine. Dr. Ali Meghoufel, who did his doctoral research work at the University of Quebec and Dr. Nathalie

Crevier-Denoix, Professor of Veterinary Medicine from France, studied the liquid interface between cells.

I asked my Morphometrix associates, "Can we use this same technology used for race horses to examine the penis?"

To find the answer, we scanned the tissue segment counts of 60 men before and after treatment, assessing the left and right cavernosum, comparing our scans with their SHIM scores. We use the scan, take the image of the ultrasound, remove the noise, and get the liquid interfaces in the tissues. We are still in the process of making sense of all our findings but our work shows a very interesting correlation with the sexual improvement in our patients. This will be one of the first objective ways to evaluate erectile dysfunction.

We wrote software to analyze the images and then access the video clips into our software. We examined the corpus cavernosum and interstitium and found that our images highly correlate with the vascular function and improved blood flow. In early 2021 our software will be functional in a report format that will be very helpful for the practitioners practicing medicine with patients with Erectile dysfunction. We can plan better treatment protocols and customized treatment options for each patient according to the pathology that we report, with the help of Morphometrix.

Three men offer examples as a way to better understand what is possible with these combined technologies.

Case Study #1

A 63-year-old male, ex-police officer, married with three children came to see me for help. He was not a smoker but suffered from diabetes mellitus type 2, hypertension, and low testosterone. He was on no beta-blockers, took hypertension medications, and ACE inhibitors. He was not on insulin, but was taking metformin for diabetes and was on testosterone replacement. He was taking Cialis and Viagra on an as-needed basis. He had no operations, no prostatectomy, and no bypass surgery.

His erectile hardness score was 3 and his SHIM score was 18. Using our Morphometrix software, his right corpus cavernosum tissue segment count measured

8.6 and his cross-sectional score was 6.7. We performed four GAINSWave treatments, each one week apart.

Four months later, his erectile hardness score was 3, SHIM score was 24, right tissue segment ultrasound score was 28.1 and the cross-sectional score was 11.7. He had that tremendous increase in his tissue segment count from 8.6 to 28.1. This correlated very well with his SHIM score increasing from 18 to 24.

Case Study #2

A 53-year-old male, retired, unmarried man with no children came to me for help. Non-smoker, his only risk factor was hypertension. He had a history of epilepsy; but that didn't contribute negatively to his sexual function. He had hypothyroidism for which he took Synthroid. He took no beta-blockers, but was taking an ACE inhibitor for his hypertension. He was taking Cialis and Viagra. His erectile hardness score was 2, and SHIM score was 10. His tissue segment count using our Morphometrix software was 18.4 and his cross-sectional score was 7.1.

We administered six GAINSWave treatments (the first three, two days apart, then a month later, the final three, one week apart) and two P-Shots®.

At his follow-up ultrasound, his erectile hardness score was 3, SHIM score 14, segment count 8.7, and cross-sectional score 8.5. That was on the right side.

Next, we applied these same steps to the left side where the tissue segment score was 47 and the cross-sectional score was 13.4. We found his left corpus cavernosum responded much better than his right corpus cavernosum! Until now, knowing this disparity between each side of his penis was nearly impossible; now we can use such knowledge to design follow up treatments with better outcomes.

Case Study #3

A 63 year-old, radio commentator, suffering from insulin-dependent diabetes, hypertension, and obesity came to see me with ED. As a smoker with the ravages of diabetes, he had already lost two toes to gangrene and amputation. After 12 GAINSWave treatments and no major improvement, we continued treatment once per month, for a total of 22 GAINSWave treatments.

Still, after 22 GAINSWave treatments, his tissue segment count was at a very low at 6.4. We decided to perform a P-Shot®. Afterwards, his segment score went up to 28. That was incredible! He had erections again and he felt fantastic. Diabetes can severely affect erectile function, so such results do not happen with everyone.

More About the Morphometrix® Interface Software

In a normal penis ultrasound, it's difficult to see what's going on. Our technology removes noise, looks at the corpus cavernosum (sponge) and the interstitial area between the sponge holes— where the blood flow occurs. We count the number of channels. If a patient has erectile dysfunction, there are fewer channels. Effective treatment increases the number of channels.

The Morphometrix interface scan is fast and does not hurt. We are using the Butterfly IQ handheld device to do our scans. We scan both corpus cavernosum in one scan. Dealing with a larger penis, we might scan the left and right in separate scans, but it only takes a minute or two to do. We scan in B mode and use the

MP4 video clip to import into our software. After importing a scan into our software we can have a report ready within 20 minutes.

In our veterinarian division our veterinarians use the software to diagnose torn tendons and follow up on the improvement of tendon repair. The cost savings and effective treatment protocols and follow up is saving the racing horse and jumping horse owners thousands of dollars a year.

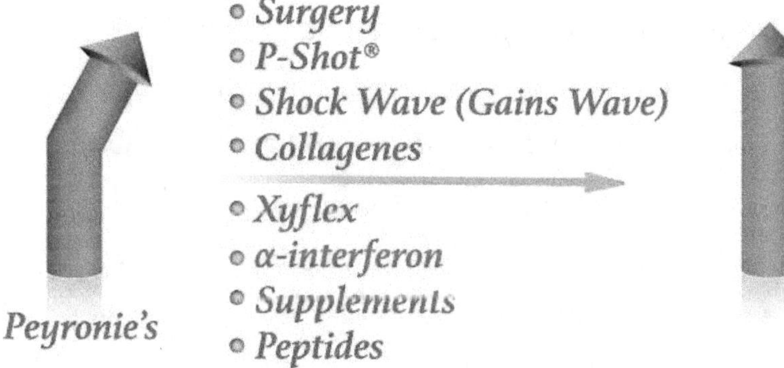

Our software shows the entire penis from beginning to end. From the base to the glans, we spot good blood flow and obstructions. The reports provide specific values for each corpus cavernosum that specifically show improvement. We can provide specific graphs of each penis ultrasound that show areas of poor blood flow. Treatment options can now be better planned by position P-Shot® applications and GAINSWave treatment protocols. Most therapies take 8 to 12 weeks to see maximum effect. We do Ultrasounds before treatment and then 8-12 weeks after the treatment protocol. If we improve with the software and a patient still has serious Erectile Dysfunction, we can focus on psychological causes and change our focus of treatment.

Optimal Body for Optimal Sex

I like to start with a panel of blood-work: CBC, electrolytes, fasting blood sugar creatinine, thyroid, LH/FSH estrogen, free testosterone and PSA. Our approach is to bring testosterone levels back to good physiological levels. We monitor CBC, Hct TSH, LH, Free Testosterone, s-DHEA and PSA and Estrogen levels every three months.

To treat younger men with low testosterone, I often use Clomid to improve free testosterone, with a combination of weight training exercises. Using injectable testosterone at an average dose of 100 milligrams per week helps bring levels back. Transdermal Testosterone is also an option instead of injectables. We have a compound pharmacy that makes gels for our patients and there are pharmaceutical companies that make transdermal products like Androgel. Testosterone pellets can also be used for men; these last up to 3 or 6 months.

For best erectile function, a man should optimize the health of his whole body. I always do a body composition, lifestyle change counseling, an exercise program, and provide designed meal plans. Our website, doc.care, is an excellent source.

 I always scan and use our software to examine the corpus cavernosum before doing a P-Shot® because it's important to get it right. As described by Dr. Runels that developed the P-Shot® positioning of the shots are very important. The ultrasound device helps us target the corpus cavernosum when injecting.

We individualize the injections. For example, with Peyronie's disease we concentrate the injections around the plaque area. The ultrasound shows where that is. For those suffering with Peyronie's disease, we also use the RestoreX stretching device from restorex.com.

Case Study #4

A 36 year-old, truck driver, married, with one child came to see me. He said he didn't need a big penis, but that his penis was asymmetric and his erection was soft. Using our Morphometrix scan, we could easily see that his left corpus cavernosum was underdeveloped in size and demonstrated fewer channels. His left side looked much worse than the right side on the scan. Treatments with P-Shot® and GAINSWave were allocated to the needed area.

Eight weeks later, there was improvement in the scan. He reported that his erections improved dramatically in symmetry and firmness; it improved his overall confidence and sexual performance that boosted his relationship with his partner.

Steps to Your Sexual Wellness

Don't be embarrassed about your situation, no matter what it may be. Most men will experience erectile dysfunction occasionally. It becomes an issue when it happens regularly. Speak up about your situation. Tell your doctor and look for the underlying etiology.

Shape up and slim down. Keeping yourself healthy will improve all aspects of your health including erectile dysfunction. Consider lifestyle changes like quitting smoking (if you smoke) and consuming less alcohol (if you drink more than 1 drink per day).

Let your doctor know if your treatment is working. There's always more that can be done. Keep in touch. Develop a follow-up plan with your doctor.

Use a ***synergy of tailor-made strategies***, but never forget that *lifestyle changes and diet are the best first-line therapy* for ED. Work with your doctor or a nutritionist to develop a meal plan that sticks.

North American Study – SWEET Study: Dr. Brandeis, a leading urologist from San Francisco, is running one of the biggest research studies on erectile dysfunction in North America.

More About Dr. Dan Botha

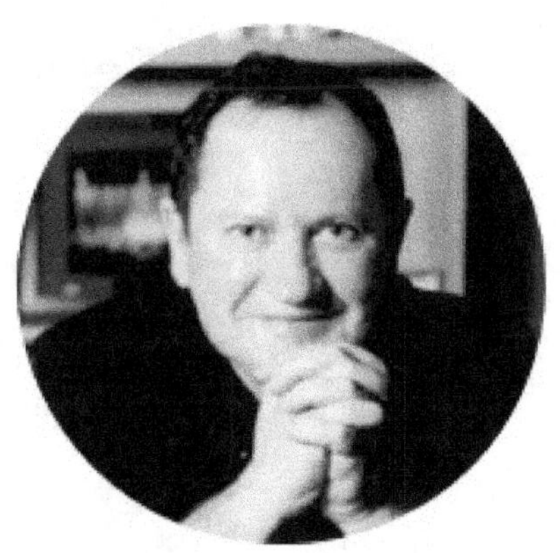

Dr. Dan Botha has been practicing medicine in Calgary for the past 25 years. In 1983 he graduated with a Bachelor of Medicine and Bachelor of Surgery from the University of the Orange Free State in Bloemfontein, South Africa. With a certification in Age Management Medicine, he has incorporated innovative treatments to improve your health and quality of life.

- Websites: DynamicHealthStudio.ca, GAINSWaveCalgary.ca, Doc.care
- Location: Calgary, Alberta, Canada
- Phone: 403-255-5868

References

1. Joice GA, Burnett AL (2016) Nonsurgical Interventions for Peyronie's Disease: Update as of 2016. World J Mens Health 34: 65-72

2. Al-Takhafi S, Al-Hatal N (2016) Peyronie's disease: a literature review on epidemiology, genetics, pathophysiology, diagnosis and work –up. Transl Andol Urol 5: 280-289

3. Chong W, Tan RB1 (2016) Injectable therapy for Peyronie's disease. Transl Androl Urol 5: 310-317.

4. Zucchi A, Costantini E, Cai T, Cavallini G, Liguori G et al. (2016) Intralesional injection of hyaluronic acid in patients affected with Peyronie's disease : Preliminary results from a prospective multicenter pilot study. Sex Med 4: 85-90

5. Ching-Shwum L, Zhong-Cheng X, Wang Z, Deng C, Huang YC, Lin G et al. (2012) Stem Cell therapy for erectile dysfunction: a critical review. Stem Cells Dev 21: 343- 351

6. Okabe K, Yamad Y, Ito K, Kohgo T, Yoshimi R et al. (2009) Injectable soft-tissue augmentation

and regenerative medicine with human mesenchymal stromal cells, platelet –rich plasma and hyaluronic acid scaffolds. Cytotherapy 11: 307-316

7. Vadalà G, Russo F, Musumeci M, D'Este M, Cattani C et al. (2016) A clinically relevant hydrogel based on hyaluronic acid and platelet rich plasma as a carrier for mesenchymal stem cells: rheological and biological characterization. J Orthop Res

8. Lana JF, Weglein A, Sampson S, Vicente EF, Huber SC et al. (2016) Randomized controlled trial comparing hyaluronic acid, platelet-rich plasma and the combination of both in the treatment of mild to moderate osteoarthritis of the knee. J Stem Cells Regen Med 12:69-78

9. Rosen RC, Cappelleri JC, Smith MD, Lipsky J, Peña BM (1999) Development and evaluation of an abridged, 5-item version of the International Index of Erectile Function (IIEF-5) as a diagnostic tool for erectile dysfunction. Int J Impot Res. 11:319-26

10. Virag R, Sussman H (2017) Evaluation of the Benefit of using a combination of autologous platelet-rich plasma and hyaluronic acid for

the treatment of Peyronie's disease. Sexual Health ISSN:2515-5660

11. Leake J, Greenberg T Textbook of Age Management Medicine Vol 1,2,3.

12. Gordon M.L The Clinical Application of Interventional Endocrinology.

Chapter 6:
Hormone Balancing for Amazing Sex & Deep Relationships
by Dr. Kimberly L. Evans

How do you know if hormone balancing is the solution you need?

A man or woman without proper hormone balance will struggle with emotions. There can be ***inappropriate anger,*** or the ***struggle to feel closeness and love,*** either can plague someone with hormone imbalances. ***Trying to think or feel your way out of hormone imbalance is like trying to think your way out of a fast heart rate if someone gave you a shot of adrenaline;*** hormones act as chemical messengers that affect the body in ways that can profoundly affect both the sexual response and personal relations. The doctor you choose should know how to expertly balance estrogen, testosterone, and progesterone, the three main hormones that help with sexual function.

Similar to many women I treat, you may not know your estrogen level is low but might be experiencing vaginal dryness, daytime hot flashes, laxity of skin, or painful intercourse. Women with low testosterone suffer from fatigue, irritability, difficulty sleeping, low libido or night sweats.

Your **progesterone** could be low. The first symptom could be irregular bleeding, mood swings, pms symptoms, headaches or insomnia. Progesterone helps balance estrogen effects within the uterus.

HORMONES

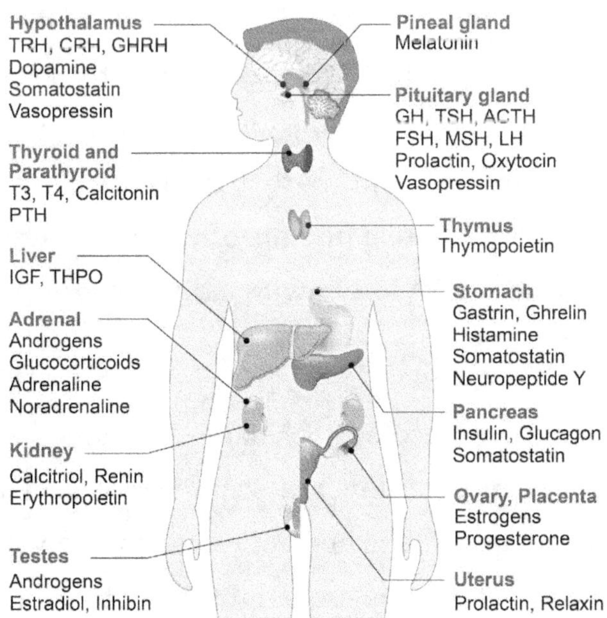

Not all hormones are created equal. Therefore, breast cancer is less prevalent in younger women. They are more hormonally balanced.

The goal of any therapy is to be balanced and as close to your own natural hormones as possible. There are different types of hormones. The right hormones delivered in a balanced fashion has shown to not increase your chance of getting breast cancer.

Look at the types of hormones your doctor offers. If they only offer synthetic hormones (not biologically identical to what the human body makes), then she may not be offering you your optimal therapy. Also, if, after following your doctor's advice, you still suffer, talk with your doctor again and let her know; don't assume there's nothing left to be done. Also, ask yourself, "Am I being properly balanced; do I need a second opinion?" Great doctors often welcome second opinions and work closely with a diverse group of expert opinions.

Though most gynecologists balance hormones, some acquire specialty training in hormone replacement. In the past, only synthetic hormones were widely available. Most doctors are taught very little about hormones in medical school. My textbook in gynecology only included a total of two pages for bioidentical hormone balancing. Most learning happens in this area after medical school both in practice, in specialty training, and by constantly reading the current research.

The BioTE method, which is backed by much research and which I follow, works well for hormone balancing. We use hormones biologically identical to what the body makes and created in an FDA-approved lab using sterile technique.

Not All Hormones Are Equal

There are three types of estrogen: estriol (E3), estradiol (E2), and estrone (E1).

E1 is usually linked to fat cells, which can cause an increased risk of breast cancer. Ensure you get estradiol that is bio-identical (chemically identical) to what comes from the human ovary; this way, side effects are minimized and therapy is optimized.

Prempro was used in a WHI (Women's Health Initiative) study and is made using synthetic estrogen from horse urine (not identical to human estrogen).

Consider the word *"Premarin" which means from a mare, or horse.* That WHI study had two arms: estrogen, then progesterone and estrogen together. The "together" study showed an increased risk of breast cancer. However, *estrogen alone showed no increased risk of breast cancer.*

Many doctors don't realize that some hormones are helpful and others are not. For example, *progestin, a type of progesterone, led to increased risk of breast cancer.* However, methyltestosterone, the type of synthetic testosterone administered orally in pill form, showed an increased risk of breast cancer. However, subcutaneous testosterone (delivered through the skin) showed no increased risk of breast cancer.

Dosing properly and subcutaneously also decreases the chance of side effects (including the risk of breast cancer), provides a longer-lasting effect, and helps you feel better. Optimized hormones— with proper dosages, types of hormones, and safer methods of delivery— lead to better results.

If you were my patient asking for hormone balancing, I would check your total testosterone level, progesterone level, and follicle-stimulating hormone level. I would also check your thyroid level. Low thyroid can lead to depression or difficulty with weight loss as well as decreased sex drive.

We check your thyroid levels: T3, T4, TSH, and thyroid peroxidase. Many of these test results may be linked to increased stress.

If you had irregular bleeding, we would focus on testosterone, thyroid and prolactin levels. Elevated follicle-stimulating hormone levels could indicate premature ovarian failure.

Just as importantly, how do you feel? Do you feel in-balance or irritable, tired, or emotionally flat?

If you have irregular bleeding, or decreased libido or difficulty with orgasm, we may check your any of the above levels.

More than 90% of patients who see us improve when we focus on micromanaging these hormones in a balanced way.

Case #1

Recently, a woman, age 48, came to see me because of a severe strain on her marriage due to her lack of sexual desire for her husband even though she deeply loved him. Counseling had not helped. Her testosterone and estradiol levels were low, and her FSH was suppressed. We discovered that her birth control pills had caused her testosterone levels to fall.

Even when people enjoy a tight relationship with most everything in place, their sexual relations will suffer if hormone levels are off. Usually, I suggest women phase out birth control pills after age thirty-five. Birth control pills increase sex hormone binding globulin (SHBG) which sucks up testosterone—lowers biologically free testosterone, leading to fatigue and decreased libido.

After stopping her birth control pills and raising her testosterone back to healthy levels, she found her sexual desire for her husband matched her emotional love for him and they became much closer.

More Signs that Your Hormones May Need Adjusting

One well documented but poorly understood phenomenon seen with women who take birth control pills can cause women to suffer with severe vaginal pain when they have sex. Unfortunately, even when these women stop taking the birth control pills, the pain can persist for months. The vagina of a young woman with this syndrome can start to respond sexually like that of a post-menopausal woman without estrogen.

Another sign of the possible need for hormone adjustment is when a woman complains of *fatigue*. Many different diseases can cause fatigue, but often women can suffer fatigue because they have a low testosterone, low thyroid, low vitamin D, or low B12 levels. These same low levels cause low sex drive and strained relationships along with the fatigue. A high prolactin level can also cause extreme fatigue.

Also, get a good OB/GYN exam to ensure nothing else is contributing to how you feel. For example, endometriosis and fibroids can lead to pain. There may also be undiagnosed ovarian tumors that lead to hormonal disorders and low sex drive.

Antidepressants and antihypertensives can cause low libido or inability to orgasm. Some people need antidepressants for emotional stability even after balancing their hormones; but, I commonly see women decrease or stop their antidepressants and feel better than ever after we get their hormones balanced. Antidepressants can also lead to weight gain, brain fog, and a "numb-to-the-world" feeling. When needed, Wellbutrin and Lexapro are usually my preferred mood stabilizers.

DHEA can help some women feel sexier and more energetic because it's a precursor to testosterone; but it's usually much less effective for sexual response than is testosterone.

What else can help you sexually? Astroglide, KY Jelly, and coconut oils can help with vaginal moisture and allow more comfortable sexual intercourse and therefore increased libido.

Also, never underestimate the power of following a healthy diet and daily exercise. Low carb meals seem to work best for weight control and energy. Reduce stress and consider massages once a week if fits your budget.

If you are obese with high E1 levels, that can activate pelvic pain. Some women can see huge improvement just by changing to a proper diet, exercising, and losing weight. Healthy eating your way to a normal body weight can lead to better estrogen balance even without taking any medicine.

Case #2

I recently saw a 23-year-old woman suffering with sexual pain from a very dry vagina— no moisture at all. ***In her case, just taking her off birth control pills and helping her with another method of birth control improved her vaginal health.***

Her blood testosterone levels increased, and her sex drive went crazy just from stopping her birth control pills. She was no longer afraid of painful intercourse or lubrication problems.

It took six months for her to go back to normal, but she did so without any medicines at all when we stopped the birth control pills.

When You Don't Feel Like Anything Is "Wrong"

Often, a woman who has lost her libido doesn't feel broken. They do not miss it. They do not feel the need to be fixed at all; and, she's absolutely right in that if she feels well, she has the option to choose to be mostly or completely asexual— that's perfectly ok.

But. before you decide to give up on sex, you may want to consider how you feel overall. Many times, my female patients will say, "I don't have a problem, but this is how my husband feels." Or "I know it is a problem with my relationship, but I don't see why I should want to have sex if I don't want to have sex."

Or some of my female patients will say, "My last doctor said, 'Get drunk and you will feel in the mood.'"

That seems sad to me that a woman would need alcohol to want to be intimate with her husband. Just one extra glass of wine every night with no other change in diet or exercise leads to an extra 10 pounds of body weight.

Before you give up on sex, consider that *low testosterone also manifests as feelings of sadness or low energy*. A dry vagina is almost unheard of before age 40 in a normal woman. You are not too old to give up on sex. I have couples in their 70's who enjoy sex 2 to 3 times per week; and that activity gives sparkle to the rest of their relationship and their lives.

It is easy to tell you it is a problem, but if you do not see sex as a problem, you will not act on it. Let's pretend intercourse is not a problem. The question becomes, "What about other areas of your life? Do you have difficulty sleeping? Do you feel angry? Are you happy with your relationships?"

Often, another sign there may be a problem is when a woman states "My friends tell me they cannot stand to be around me at times." Or, the woman may say, "I'm yelling at my husband. I love him dearly. While I'm yelling, I wonder why I'm yelling. I can't stop."

When the woman feels better, her health is better, her sex drive grows, relationships can deepen. Her husband and children feel better because the woman of the house feels better. Her better health and better sex can help reunite and save relationships.

Three Types of Women Who See Me

Sometimes, treating sexual issues gives women the strength to leave a relationship, instead of saving it. The women I treat usually fall into one of three groups:

- **The first group:** she feels broken but has a wonderful husband. He is healthy with a great job. He may exercise regularly and has no sexual issues. When she gets hormonally balanced, the marriage problem is solved. They live happily ever after.
- **Group two:** she's 40 pounds overweight, no sex drive, he has three girlfriends on the side and treats her like dirt. She improves and gets her mojo back, leaves her husband, and is happier without the husband and with her better health.
- **Group three:** the husband suffers with obesity and diabetes and the woman is not healthy. They love each other. She gets well and she's disturbed because now she doesn't want any other man. She loves her husband; but now, he

can't keep up with her newfound health and high sex drive. So, she becomes very frustrated but does not want to leave. Therefore, the following week he is coming in to see me too.

The first couple is healthy and they live happily ever after. The second couple splits up immediately; and there's nothing I can do. The final group requires the husband's participation. It helps if I can check her partner's hormones and show those levels. I explain the health benefits: healthier heart, more muscle, increased clarity of thinking, and more strength. In the end, they are both happy with a renewed outlook on their marriage.

Case #3

One of my favorite couples comes to mind. The woman was pelleted. An hour later, her husband called and said, "It's time for MY pellet." He knows she will run off and leave him (libido-wise) if he doesn't catch up. He wants to be at her level.

I have couples who learned to take better care of themselves, in general. They know that overall their health depends on it. That is the most important thing. Sex is a bonus, but health improvement, strength, bones, and brain, make a person sexier.

A patient came to see me once, looking wonderful from head to toe, but she was crying. She looked like she stepped out of a magazine. ***She was overcompensating for feeling broken on the inside*** and I see this a lot. She was not herself on the insider. By adjusting her hormones, many women will get what they need to feel normal again, regain confidence and feel better.

That will show from the inside out!

Preventing Breast Cancer

If you are not on the right progesterone, you can have an increased chance of irregular bleeding. The progesterone hormone is dominant in the second half of your cycle. Good progesterone can balance you out: give you better sleep, give more energy in the morning and reduce irregular bleeding.

Bad progesterone can lead to increased weight gain, bloating, and sadness. We make sure to use the right type of hormone for the right patient. Let's pretend you were my patient and asked about the progesterone-only Depo-Provera shot. If you were 20 years old and wanted to prevent pregnancy, I think it is an excellent choice to have a birth control you did not have to think about outside of 4 times per year. However, after 40, we would have more of an in depth conversation about potential side effects since it can increase appetite and lead to weight gain.

Progesterone can be synthetic or natural. Natural progesterone is made from wild yam. I prefer micronized progesterone, like Prometrium. This hormone has steadier, even absorption. One study showed progesterone has an anti-proliferative effect on breast cancer and leukemia cells[1].

If you are a woman without a uterus, you do not need progesterone unless you have difficulty sleeping or a history of endometriosis. We balance everything else. If you are a woman with a uterus, we must use progesterone to balance out estrogen and prevent irregular bleeding.

When an older or perimenopausal woman needs progesterone, micronized progesterone is usually the best and safest type. Another study showed that women experience greater sexual satisfaction, improved quality of life and have fewer side effects with micronized progesterone. Many of the negative side effects can occur when a patient switches from Progestin to progesterone[2,3].

Bioidentical progesterone showed a 30% reduction in sleep problems, 50% reduction in anxiety, 60% reduction in depression, 25% reduction in menstrual bleeding and 30% improvement in sexual function compared to non-bioidentical progesterone.

If you are a woman concerned about breast cancer and you do not want to be on hormones, my question to you would be, "What concerns have you had?" The answer is usually, "My doctor told me about the WHI study." The way that the study was interpreted by many providers is not correct. Many women were taken off their hormones all together due to a fear of increased risk of breast cancer. However, when the study was dissected and broken down, it showed some flaws in the interpretation. The idea that estradiol was not safe is flawed. Our ovaries make estradiol. In fact the estrogen alone arm showed no increased risk for breast cancer. ***The culprit was the type of progesterone in Prempro***. Many ladies halted hormone treatment, but then returned with time when they realized and were properly informed on the benefits of cardiovascular health, sexual function, cognitive function and bone strength.

If you are afraid of breast cancer, I take a proper history to determine any increased risk above the general population and then customize your dosing for your total regimen.

Some ladies may need testosterone instead of estrogen. We can administer progesterone as a troche (with lower side effects) that dissolves under your tongue. If you have trouble sleeping, oral capsules are better.

Testosterone & Pellet Therapy

Pellet therapy allows us to customize our dosing to you. The goal of any hormone therapy is to maximize benefits without causing adverse side effects. The key driving factor is for you to feel better and appreciate the beneficial effects that hormone therapy provides. Even a slight bit of acne or abnormal hair growth is a reason to readjust.

It is important to increase energy levels. Increasing your energy can enable you to exercise more. That can decrease comorbidities (diabetes and high blood pressure) and improve your cardiovascular health.

Testosterone can help women feel stronger in your muscles and bones, especially if you have a family history of osteoporosis. Increasing your testosterone can increase your lean muscle mass, thereby leading to weight loss. Other ladies may not be sexually active but enjoy their cognitive ability to focus, remember, or be more intellectually productive at work and at home.

The breast has estrogen receptors. A healthy adequate dose of testosterone can downregulate the estrogen receptors thereby decreasing your chance of getting breast cancer. There are testosterone receptors in the vagina and adding testosterone in that area can increase blood flow and make intercourse more comfortable.

Testosterone can decrease muscle aches, increase flexibility, and decrease inflammation. When you move better, you're in a better mood.

After checking labs and determining proper dosage, we administer hormones. We recheck your labs after 5 to 6 weeks, verifying levels are normal, and ensuring you feel well. If you feel okay and your levels are normal, we keep you where you are. If you are not feeling well enough or you want to increase libido, we can readminister and give you a boost of hormones to balance you out.

You are much more than lab results; you are a patient with symptoms in need of results. Some patients are optimally dosed between 150 to 250. Others do not feel anything until they are closer to 300. Still others experience acne breakouts above 250. Every patient is different. Customized dosing is so important in balancing hormones, minimizing side effects and helping patients feel better.

We were recently nominated and won awards for best in hormone balancing in 2019 and 2020 by Living Magazine. This is best for our county in Sugar Land, Texas.

We place pellets every 3 to 4 months in women and 4 to 6 months in men in the subcuticular area of the buttocks. After determining the proper dose, it takes approximately 3 minutes to pellet a woman and 10 minutes to pellet a man.

These techniques are done in sterile conditions. The incision site is less than a width of the top of an eraser. Pellets are the size of tic-tacs. They are spread out throughout the tissue. As they slowly dissolve, testosterone is released. We can get steady-state optimized levels.

Estrogen

We sometimes use estrogen pellets along with testosterone. Some doctors use testosterone pellets that are not BioTE, requiring oral estrogen. To me, It's a disservice to have to take a pill every day when it can be in the form of a pellet.

After that basic step of checking your levels, we might consider estrogen therapy if you complain about hot flashes, dry skin, or a dry vagina. Low levels can also decrease collagen. This can lead to cellulite and saggy skin, which we see many times.

If your bones are weak, you may benefit from estrogen therapy for estradiol. Estradiol is secreted from the ovaries. Estrogen has only a few negative side effects, but if you get too much estrogen, you could experience breast tenderness and moodiness.

Many gynecologists are fine providing vaginal estrogen cream to women who survived breast cancer. It helps keep the vagina healthy, keeps levels low, and keeps local tissue healthy without changing the bloodstream as much as oral therapy. This is a great option for a woman terrified of breast cancer when non hormonal options are not enough.

A proper well woman exam is important. Get evaluated with a thorough breast exam and regular mammograms. As long as your mammogram is normal, there's no indication to avoid estrogen therapy.

Most people feel the results of hormone therapy in 5 to 14 days. We bring the patient back 5 to 6 weeks later and check hormones again. Some ladies have low levels but feel fantastic. They do not need tweaking.

Others tell me their levels are acceptable but could feel better. A patient like that can use a hormone adjustment.

This is the benefits of pellet therapy. I have many doses to adjust to help customize the dose and help the patient feel better.

O-Shot® (Platelet-Rich Plasma) and Radio Frequency

O-Shot® and radiofrequency can help with sexual dysfunction. We can also add hormonal balancing with the O-Shot® to enhance sensation and your ability to have an orgasm. Hormones can help restore moisture, increase blood flow and thereby increase sensation. Radiofrequency, increases lubrication and helps build collagen. This can decrease laxity thereby increasing sensation.

We can perform the O-Shot® procedure and hormones at the same time. *I can perform radio frequency on the vagina, surgery, or Emsella.*

I have written a research paper on Emsella, which helps with urinary incontinence and sexual dysfunction.

Emsella improves orgasm and sexual satisfaction. It's like doing 11,000 Kegels in a 28-minute session. Anything that can help the pelvis with grip, feeling, and to decrease uncomfortable urinary problems, helps to enhance sexual satisfaction.

Radio frequency is great if a woman can't feel her partner, or has increased laxity— perhaps due to childbirth or age. Radio frequency helps enhance and increase collagen in the area and leads to overall enhanced sexual function.

As a board certified gynecologist nearing 20 years of experience, I am well trained in all the feminine organs: the uterus, tubes, ovaries, cervix, vagina, and vulva. Anything that goes wrong in those areas can lead to sexual dysfunction. If you don't feel adequate, see a doctor who specializes in that area. This differentiates me from an average dermatologist who may perform hormone therapy or be doing these vaginal procedures.

Starting Point

I start with a basic workup to discover if anything is organically wrong, preventing you from having orgasms. If you have pain during sex, is it pain in the vagina or in a different location? I start with a good workup to ensure there's nothing wrong with the uterus.

Fibroids, masses, tumors, or ovarian cysts can lead to pelvic pain and subsequent dysfunction. Minimally invasive or more involved surgeries are options to fix your problem and help you feel normal. I can treat a variety of things such as abnormal pap smears, major surgery to remove fibroids and minimally invasively treatment for irregular bleeding. I can perform surgery to tighten your vagina if there is too much laxity.

I talk to you and listen to how you feel. Perhaps you have a healthy vagina, but can't feel anything during intercourse. If you birthed multiple large babies, you could have a stretched-out vagina. Air could get trapped in that area leading to abnormal sounds during intercourse or embarrassing loss of urine.

Irregular bleeding can be caused by something structurally wrong or hormonally wrong. Do you have problems with defecation or constipation? Those could be symptoms of laxity in the vaginal wall. After a thorough exam, I look for laxity in the upper or lower wall of your vagina— or any prolapse in the cervix or vagina.

Imagine the upper or lower vagina tightened, repaired, restored to a previous state. We correct some of what you feel or don't feel. Consider possible aesthetic improvements, such as correcting an extremely long labia, which can drag or make intercourse uncomfortable. That can be corrected with a labiaplasty. Moles or abnormal growths in that area can lead to lack of self confidence. It is important to have a doctor with the ability to address and treat multiple concerns.

Genital Mismatch

A man loses 50% of his penis endothelium by the time he's 65 years old; and, a woman who delivers vaginally may see an increase in her vaginal laxity; so, his penis is shrinking and her vagina's growing. They still love each other, but their genitals become mismatched.

Another situation: sometimes the woman has previously had a vaginal tightening procedure and she's married to "King Kong." She could be genetically small or have had surgery for a neoplasia. Now, they love each other but suffer with a genital mismatch.

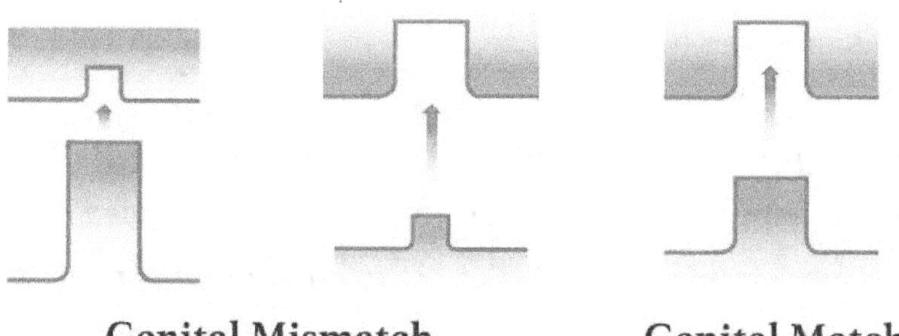

Genital Mismatch can cause decreased sexual pleasure or pain.

A good history (physical exam) is important. Women generally don't offer that information, and men definitely don't offer that information.

If a woman complains of laxity, I ask, "What penis size are you working with at home?" I lay out vaginal dilators in different sizes. Sometimes she says, "I have problems with laxity." I line up the dilators and say, "Show me what you're working with. I don't want to over tighten." That's important. I can attempt to customize her vagina for her lover's fit.

There are those who criticize us by claiming we make a woman feel insecure about her vagina after she's given birth. As if the only goal is to satisfy her husband, give him more pleasure. It's also about her having more pleasure, especially after vaginally birthing eight-pound babies. It's not only about pleasing her husband.

If she loves her husband, why wouldn't she want him to be happy too? It's about how she can have pleasure by feeling what's there. We try to customize her surgery not only for her partner to feel better, but so she has more pleasure, and she feels better.

When having these discussions with women, I say, "Tell me what you want." It begins with her. Where do those next steps in improving your sex life begin? What do you want and need? By starting with what is affecting her the most important because we are more complex. Many things can interfere with our sexual satisfaction and ability to climax.

Steps to Your Sexual Wellness

1. If you notice vaginal dryness, loss of libido, low energy, difficulty sleeping, or vaginal bleeding, talk to a doctor that specializes in hormone balancing. That physician should know how to balance estrogen, testosterone, and progesterone. These are three main hormones that help with sexual dysfunction.

2. If your doctor offers therapy and you don't feel right, ask if you are being properly balanced. Imbalanced hormones can lead to several negative effects on your well-being.

3. Speak to a doctor about long-term unexplained symptoms, especially those that cause pain, discomfort, or interfere with everyday activities. Continue to keep regular gynecology appointments for your overall health.

More About Dr. Kimberly L. Evans

Dr. Kimberly L. Evans is a specialist in women's healthcare, sexual health, and aesthetic treatments. She is a board-certified OB/GYN with nearly 20 years of experience. Recognized as the "female orgasm doctor" for her expertise in resolving sexual dysfunction, she has spent her career helping women and men be healthier, feel sexier, and live happier.

- Website: SugarLandMedSpa.com
- Location: Sugar Land, Texas, USA
- Phone: 281-277-7721

References

1. Formby B, Wiley TS. Progesterone inhibits growth and induces apoptosis in breast cancer cells: inverse effects on Bcl-2 and p53. Ann Clin Lab Sci. 1998;28(6):360-369.

    https://pubmed.ncbi.nlm.nih.gov/9846203/

2. Maxson WS, Hargrove JT. Bioavailability of oral micronized progesterone. Fertil Steril. 1985;44(5):622-626.

    https://pubmed.ncbi.nlm.nih.gov/4054341/

3. Ryan N, Rosner A. Quality of life and costs associated with micronized progesterone and medroxyprogesterone acetate in hormone replacement therapy for nonhysterectomized, postmenopausal women. Clin Ther. 2001;23(7):1099-1115. doi:10.1016/s0149-2918(01)80094-1

    https://pubmed.ncbi.nlm.nih.gov/11519773/

Chapter 7:
Recover Your Sex Life
After Prostate Cancer
with Dr. Ramesh Kumar

When I was 14 years old, my Dad died. Afterwards, my brother-in-law took over the support and care of our home. He became a deserving hero to me at a time when I needed a solid role model.

Then, within a year of my Father's death, my-brother-in-law was diagnosed with testicular cancer and died of it. *Even as a teenager, I noticed that he was treated horribly by the chemotherapy doctors. His mistreatment horrified and angered me.*

So, after that incident, I vowed that I would become a cancer doctor and treat every person who came to me for help with much better than "average" skill and respect. I've spent the rest of my life doing my best to keep that vow. As part of keeping that vow, *I became convinced that taking excellent care of people who battle cancer must involve paying attention to their sexual function and relations.*

With prostate cancer, often doctors assume that their patient's erectile dysfunction (ED) is caused by chemotherapy, radiation, or surgery given for the cancer. Rather than assume the ED is from the prostate surgery, it is best to take a step back and see if something predated the prostate cancer.

For example, if you came to me for help with your sexual function in your recovery from prostate cancer treatment, I would start by looking at your metabolic profile. Many people have metabolic syndrome with a borderline hemoglobin A1C, but they do not yet have full blown diabetes.

Let's explore other *strategies to help recover full blown sexual function even after being attacked by prostate cancer.*

Prostate Cancer Survivors Should Still Enjoy Sex

Around 170,000 men are diagnosed with prostate cancer every year; and, tragically, 35,000 of those men will die from it. But, most men struck by prostate cancer do not die from it; they die of something else.

I personally treated at least 500 people for their cancer, one-on-one, every year for the past 20 years. That is a total of 10,000 people. When I treat them, I always inquire about their social situation and search for other factors, like sexual relations, that are affected by their cancer diagnosis. I attended Harvard medical school to learn about the interaction of mind-body medicine. The impact is enormous.

When my patients first heard the news about their diagnosis of prostate cancer from their urologist, here is what they often say they were thinking:

- "It's like I was kicked in the balls."
- "It hurts so much, not just physically, but emotionally."

- "It's as if my manhood has been taken out."

Can you relate? Have you heard bad news such as this, or know a friend or family member with prostate cancer? You do not need to feel helpless.

As an example, as part of my evaluation, I can look at your metabolic profile, psychological, and social factors (i.e., cigarette smoking) that contribute to erectile dysfunction before and after prostate cancer. Patients are usually focused on their diet at first, but there's much more to consider.

The Curable Population

The population that most needs serious attention with erectile dysfunction are patients with prostate cancer, and those who are curable. Men diagnosed with stage 1 and stage 2 prostate cancer are extremely treatable. The cure rate with radiation or surgery is exceptionally high.

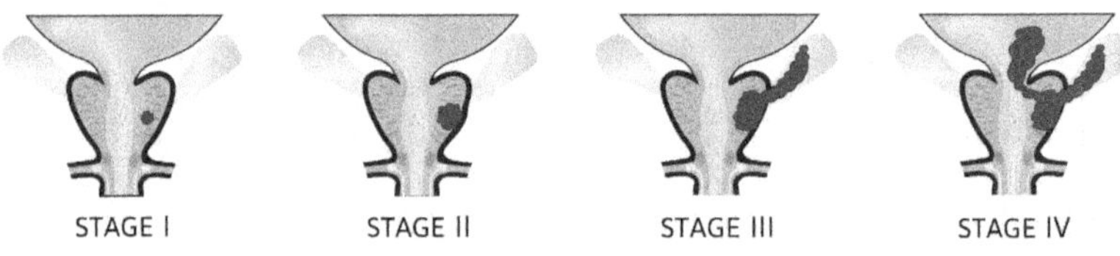

When a patient has advanced prostate cancer, we sometimes must reduce testosterone levels. The population I'm looking at are patients with a decent level of testosterone, erectile dysfunction, and a long lifespan.

Patients who undergo radiation and surgery **do not always need androgen deprivation therapy,** but it's good to know the testosterone levels to show where you are.

There's a controversy on whether we need to replace testosterone in the face of prostate cancer. Most people assume that in all cases, it is not acceptable.

But, some men, after treatment for prostate cancer, can benefit greatly from testosterone treatment.

If you came to me to treat your erectile dysfunction, I would start by carefully measuring your LH, FSH, prolactin levels, liver function, and sex hormone binding globulin levels. Then by strategically tailoring replacement of hormones based on symptoms and keeping the prostate cancer beaten back, we can see sexual relations and well-being function on very high levels— even after the prostate cancer treatment.

Most men have never had an erectile dysfunction evaluation, even before prostate surgery or radiation. They might have tested PSA or testosterone levels, but often no one ever checks important baseline hormone levels.

When a urologist sends a patient to me for radiation, before doing anything to treat the cancer, we check your erectile dysfunction score.

I especially enjoy treating men over age 70 with extremely high surgical risks. If you are under age 70, we advise surgery unless you have heart issues or your cancer is medically inoperable.

Counseling

Part of my strategies in the treatment of prostate cancer include using the huge power of the mind-body connection— including the understanding that your situation is curable. I know how to be very truthful and provide hope at the same time. Many patients are "stuck in the darkness" based on discouraging advice from others.

Their last physician might have said, in essence, "This is difficult to get rid of. You'll die."

But, anything is possible. The goal is to get rid of the cancer, ease suffering, and put men back on track with their relationships.

Consider the obesity epidemic. Most men with prostate cancer are stressed and so eat more and gain weight. That's their way of de-stressing. They also lose sleep. Then, the lack of sleep worsens their testosterone levels and contributes to erectile dysfunction. This downward cascade of health is triggered by this initial conversation the man with prostate cancer has with his urologist.

We often help boost the cancer treatment by providing easy diet recommendations. I developed a diet program called "The Prolonged Diet" that works well to help boost a man's health and normalize his weight while we defeat prostate cancer.

It may be helpful to think briefly about the Prolonged Diet to better understand how thinking about overall health can help defeat cancer and restore sexual relations.

The Prolonged Diet & Tiny Habits

If you're undergoing radiation (or any type of treatment for cancer), you must be cathartic— get rid of everything that slows the body's ability to fight disease and win. For the overweight, losing weight definitely helps with the battle. Stored visceral fat is not just a storage of energy; visceral fat acts like a gland that can secrete health-harming chemicals and hormones. You can start to rid your body of visceral fat and restore optimal health by changing one tiny habit— this is your starting point to build a new healthy way of life that helps create a healthier body.

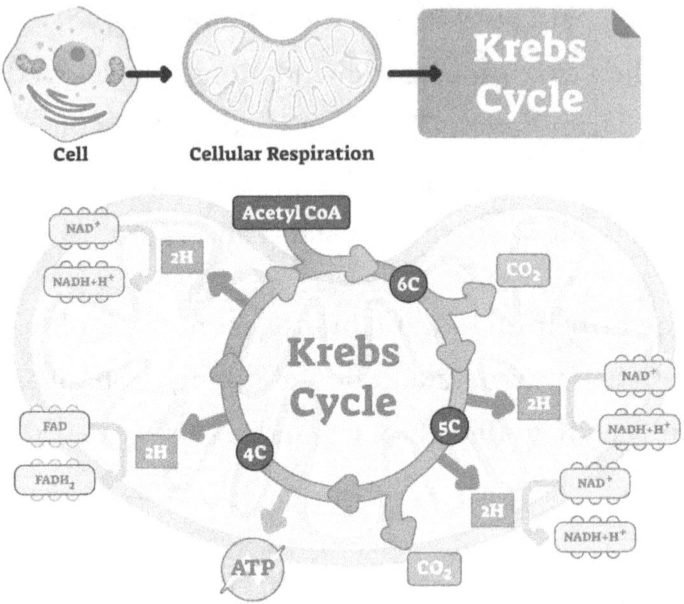

You can actually get into ketosis with The Prolonged Diet during the treatment phase of your battle with prostate cancer. This diet goes after visceral fat rather than subcutaneous fat. It is a healthy fat loss. Strong scientific research supports healthy stem cell regeneration and age reversal benefits from this diet.

I understand that diet, weight loss, and age management may not be the highest priority right now for most people with prostate cancer; defeating cancer is. However, lifestyle modification, like a healthy eating plan that is doable, can get you to a quicker recovery in months instead of years.

Another plan that I enjoy is intermittent fasting. I eat one meal every day, subjecting my body to a 16-hour fast over 24 hours. Most people love that plan after their body gets used to it.

The excellent health that defeats cancer and brings a speedy recovery (including better sex) **begins with changing daily habits.** When you wake up, what do you do? You go to the bathroom, brush your teeth, and perhaps make coffee. One step subconsciously leads to the next. These are built-in habits that can be triggered by the environment and by other habits.

One very easy and effective strategy to better health is to use an existing habit as a trigger to introduce a new habit. Let's say you want to begin flossing your teeth. As soon as you put your toothbrush down, reach for dental floss, and only floss one tooth. Link (or trigger) that existing habit into your new habit.

Very Important: Your new habit should only last five seconds, so your brain doesn't agonize about it. Floss that one tooth, then celebrate. You're anchoring it: connecting something you already do to some new five-second activity. **Then, for an entire week, repeat this 5 second behavior triggered by another habit.**

How does this strategy apply to your diet? Let's say you want to reduce your sugar intake. Remove anything sugary from your refrigerator. Make it hard to reach. When you feel the urge for sugar, eat a vegetable for 5 seconds.

As an example, imagine that now, upon opening your refrigerator door, your existing habit is to reach for a piece of candy. Instead, take that candy from the refrigerator and move it to the garage (so it's more difficult to grab). Place carrots in the same location.

When you open that refrigerator door, you're triggered to reach for candy. Instead, grab a carrot and take a bite. Celebrate that small win to solidify it. Repeat this every time you open the refrigerator door.

You can apply this same logic even if you start a weight loss system such as Weight Watchers or Nutrisystem. Redirect your habits and stick with a plan for at least five days.

We encourage families to change their eating plans together. A husband and wife might begin a new diet even if they don't suffer from obesity. Healthy eating offers many benefits other than weight loss — especially when fighting cancer.

Anxiety, Depression, Meditation & Brain Photobiomodulation

Another strategy to improve health when fighting cancer is meditation. Just 5 to 20 minutes of meditation can down-regulate your sympathetic system and up-regulate your parasympathetic system— leading to tranquility and to improved health and cancer fighting ability.

In 2014, Harvard Medical School ran a study[1] of randomized patients off the street. They ran MRI brain scans to get a baseline, provided a questionnaire about their stress levels, then told half of the group to meditate 20 minutes per day for eight weeks. The other half was told not to meditate, and instead continue with normal behavior.

After eight weeks, those patients returned for a new questionnaire to report stress levels and received new functional MRI scans of the brain. The result was a massive increase in gray matter from those who applied basic meditation, 20 minutes per day, for eight weeks.

You do not need to travel to the Himalayas to experience a massive level of change, productivity, creativity, and reduction in your stress. It can be a simple 15-minute process. Meditation actually does change the physical structure of your brain. Psychologically, meditation can solve many of your problems.

As part of our strategy with those fighting cancer, we use a brain photobiomodulation helmet that comfortably goes on your head like a science fiction hat and shoots low-level lasers at specific parts of your brain. It takes 20 minutes and refurbishes the whole brain. I discovered this while learning about acupuncture at Harvard Medical School. Vight manufactures the laser cap helmet for $2,000.

Better Energy Even with Cancer

Energy is not just for feeling good. The body needs energy both to be well and to fight cancer. ATP is the currency of energy in your body. When there is inflammation in your brain and body, it reduces ATP production because there is an enzyme in the citric acid cycle that affects the electron transport mechanism.

Photobiomodulation lasers activate that enzyme to jumpstart ATP production and increase those levels. That contributes to your sense of well-being and helps you escape depression. I prefer this approach instead of medications like antidepressants and drugs, which can create more problems, including erectile dysfunction.

This method only takes 20 minutes per day. Wear the cap while reading a book, watching TV, or driving. There's a science behind it. Active studies are suggesting it even helps to reverse dementia.

We also have a "whole body photobiomodulation" system from NovaThor, which works well if you experience aches and pains from a chronic fatigue syndrome. It is similar to a tanning bed, but it produces laser light. You lie down for 15 minutes and walk out feeling like a million bucks with no pain. Some Olympic athletes in the 2016 Olympics attributed winning results to this bed, which they shipped from Seattle to Rio de Janeiro for the Olympics.

Be sure and watch your sleep. Changing sleep patterns are a big indicator of your mental health.

Men can be macho. If your spouse is sitting next to you in my office, you would probably not want to admit weakness. If I asked you about your sleep patterns, your spouse might interject, "He tosses and turns. He doesn't sleep well."

That gives me a trigger to understanding your situation. I can begin a conversation with you and your partner, or individually, only with you. You are looking for hope and truth to get you to peace.

Many supplements help with sleep, including glycine, pregnenolone, zinc, and magnesium. Melatonin may help, but it leaves me groggy. Sleep apnea could be an issue related to obesity and metabolic syndrome issues. That is where a pulmonologist can assist.

If you've been diagnosed with prostate cancer, focus on your health. You may feel "kicked in the butt" by prostate cancer. You are more aware of your mortality, aware of how your body is reacting, and you are motivated to create change. *If you feel that you will do anything to ensure the cancer does not return, this volition can be a wonderful help to your path to your best physical and mental health and to your improved sexual relations.*

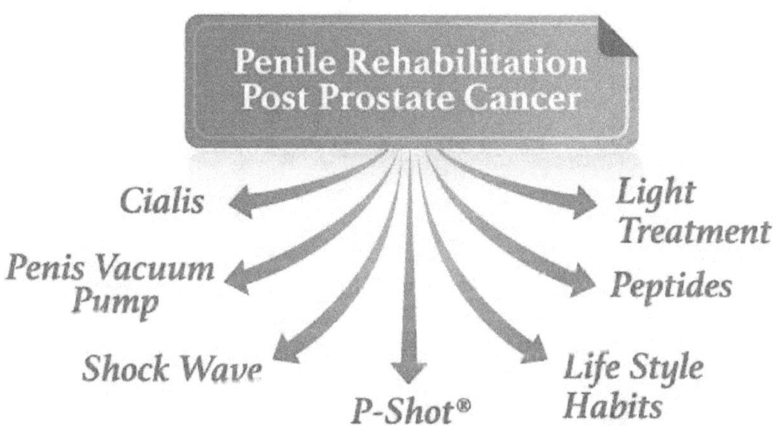

A synergistic strategy for post prostate cancer penile rehabilitation.

I'm available to every patient 24/7. I sometimes get weird calls in the middle of the night. Patients can reach me directly at my cell phone number. I like to provide reassurance, and (if you're my patient) I am here with you every step of the way.

I do not want to overwhelm you with too many options or ideas; that's my job to know. I simply want you to know that there are many options in the aftercare of cancer treatment that are available to you. All of these strategies can help reduce your stress level and shorten your recovery time.

Let's go over a few more ideas that can help.

Radiation (& Other) Strategies To Kill Cancer and Save Health

The effects of radiation on erectile dysfunction will worsen over the first two years compared to having a prostate removed through surgery, where erectile dysfunction (due to nerve damage) occurs right away and improves over two years.

If you do have surgery for prostate cancer, I can apply shockwave therapy to the penis within 3-4 months after you are done with side effects of the surgery and have recuperated from nerve damage. New data shows you might need shockwave and the P-Shot® procedure earlier than three months following surgery.

Let's pretend your prostate was removed a year ago. Before taking any action, I would ask about your sexual function. My goal is to address your individual issues and overall health. We would then likely start with Viagra or Cialis. If that fails, we would consider Gainswave and a P-Shot® procedure (PRP injected in a specific way).

If you underwent radiation treatment for your prostate cancer, we might monitor your sexual functioning over time and adjust the treatment according to how your body changes.

There are several ways of doing radiation for prostate cancer: the simplest and most effective one, with the longest track record, and available in all countries, is intensity-modulated radiation. Compare this to proton therapy, whose cure rates are no different than regular external beam radiation, and creates more damage, which might impact your sexual function. Very few locations still perform proton therapy for prostate cancer.

Regular radiation is like a bullet, and it produces bullet-like damage. A proton beam is like shooting a cannonball. You do not need to use a cannonball to destroy a rat; you need a good bullet that's expertly aimed by an expert radiation oncologist.

Some providers discuss seed placement, where radioactive seeds are placed inside the prostate, reducing the damage in the surrounding tissue. That provider must be extremely well-trained to avoid severe side effects and to effectively kill the cancer cells.

Radiation has a good track record of controlling these cancers. The treatment lasts for 8-9 weeks, five days a week. This simple form of radiation is available in any community setting. You do not need to travel thousands of miles.

By stretching the radiation treatment across 8-9 weeks, we have time to monitor you, course-correct, and figure out dosing. There's no emergency. It is targeted with our software, making it difficult to make mistakes when treating prostate cancer with radiation.

After radiation, erectile function can decline over the following two years. Many patients begin Viagra and Cialis soon after radiation. If your erectile dysfunction advances, where Viagra or Cialis was working 2-3 weeks ago but are no longer effective, we can consider Gainswave and a series of P-Shot® procedures.

We know the vasculogenic effect of radiation. Radiation cuts off the blood supply in the perineal area. GAINSwave (or Shockwave therapy) breaks up those blood clots going into the penis. It regenerates blood vessels and nerves.

If I had all the power in the world, I would require insurance companies to include this treatment in penile rehab post-prostate cancer treatment. Part of that rehabilitation process can be daily Cialis, a vacuum pump, Shockwave therapy, and P-Shot® procedures.

There's a special supplement called Affirm, part of the Shockwave therapy protocols, which increases levels of nitric oxide. I suggest 0.1cc twice a week. It functions better after completing Shockwave therapy and P-Shot®. With this maintenance plan, you come to my office once a month, and you use it at home.

A peptide (insulin is a peptide) is a chain of amino acids in a particular sequence. When your body's insulin level drops, you get diabetes. Insulin (a peptide) corrects diabetes. Sequences of amino acids provide us with different peptides that work in different parts of the body for different situations. Researchers are now creating a peptide "shot" for depression and one for anxiety. I often use peptides to help with sex in men after the prostate cancer treatment. One of those peptides in particular is very effective to increase libido— PT141 (Bromelain); but, I use other peptides with great success with men recovering from prostate cancer.

Shockwave Therapy

Acoustic waves break up kidney stones using a process called lithotripsy. That same principle can be used to help men recover from prostate cancer. The treatment is very easy and can be done with a 20 minute visit twice a week, for a total of six sessions.

We use numbing cream and then a sound-wave gun to produce shockwaves that travel through the penis. A bullet in this gun hits a diaphragm. It produces sound waves that clean out diseased blood vessels clogged with plaque buildup that cause poor circulation in the penis. This process brings new blood into the tissue which improves erection. The *shock waves also propagate the regeneration of new nerve tissue.*

This whole process works in great synergy with the Priapus Shot® (P-Shot®) procedure. The shockwave therapy opens *new "highways"* in your penis. The P-Shot® creates more lanes. Both together create new blood flow and better erections after prostate cancer.

Next Steps to Your Sexual Wellness

1. Get an erectile dysfunction workup. Test all appropriate levels. Get the full picture and don't limit yourself to just one or two tests.
2. Find a way to practice meditation in some form for 20 minutes a day to manage your stress and mental health.
3. Think about cutting down or eliminating sugar. Any change you want to make in your life, especially with diet, happens through changing tiny habits.
4. Know your options following chemotherapy, radiation, or prostate surgery— including shockwave treatment, platelet-rich plasma (Priapus Shot®), and peptides like PT141 Bromelain.

More About Dr. Ramesh Kumar

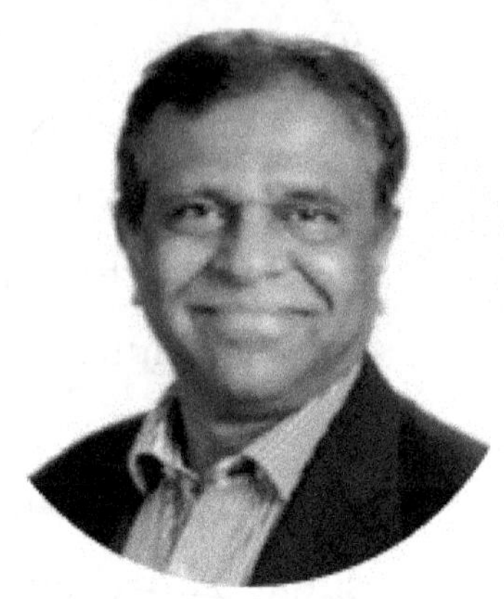

Ramesh Kumar, MD, offers his patients unmatched expertise at the practice locations in Port Saint Lucie, Palm Beach, and Palm Beach Gardens, Florida. Dr. Kumar strives to deliver exceptional patient care and believes in the value of holistic, integrative medicine. He is proud to share his skills with patients seeking alternative treatments. Dr. Kumar aims to help his patients find solutions, even if other treatments have failed. He looks forward to helping patients in his community find lasting pain relief and enjoy a more active lifestyle.

- **Website:** LifeWellMD.com
- **Location:** Palm Beach, Florida, USA
- **Phone:** 561-330-5146

References

1. Corliss, J. (2014). Mindfulness meditation may ease anxiety, mental stress. Harvard Medical School, Harvard Health Publishing.

215

Epilogue: Now What?

Now that you've made it through this book, *did you make an appointment to discuss your plans with your physician, sex therapist, pelvic floor therapist, nutritionist, personal trainer, pulmonologist, oncologist, family physician, or someone else on your health care team?*

Only by doing does knowing become valuable.

I hope, in addition to visiting the people on your health care team, that you *make plans to continue to find more help and motivation* in at least *all of the following places*:

- The *websites of each of the authors* of the chapters of this book (found at the end of each chapter).
- SexualWellnessBook.com
- OShot.com
- PriapusShot.com
- OrgasmSystem.com

Sex is an art that's never completely mastered.

Health is a gift that's made stronger with daily routines that care for that gift. I'm praying for your best wellness, sexual and otherwise, and that this book may have been some help to you and to those whom you love.

Sincerely,

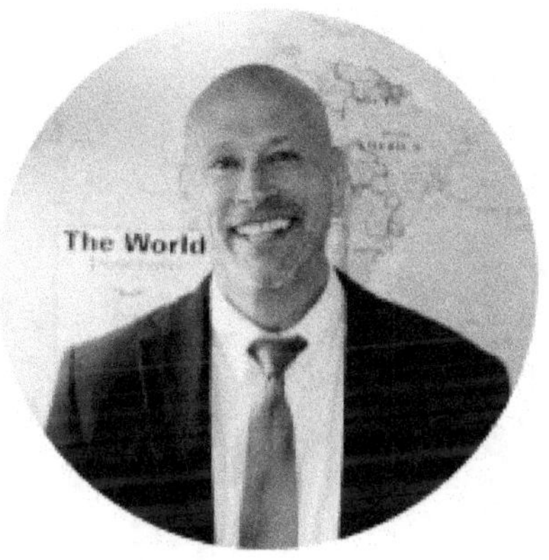

Charles Runels, MD

Fairhope, AL

November 2020

Leave a review on Amazon: SexualWellnessBook.com/amazon
Free gift from Dr. Charles Runels: SexualWellnessBook.com/gift